I0697148

Beneath the Rhythm

Living Courageously with Congestive Heart Failure

CADE STEVENSON

Copyright © 2023 by Cade Stevenson

All rights reserved. No part of this publication may be reproduced, distributed, or transmitted in any form or by any means, including photocopying, recording, or other electronic or mechanical methods, without the prior written permission of the publisher, except in the case of brief quotations embodied in critical reviews and certain other noncommercial uses permitted by copyright law.

This book and its contents are protected by copyright. No part of the material protected by this copyright may be reproduced or utilized in any form, electronic or mechanical, including photocopying, recording, or by any information storage and retrieval system, without written permission from the author

and publisher.

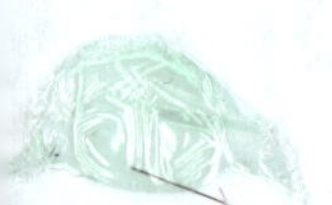

Introduction

In the realm of the human experience, stories have a remarkable ability to captivate our hearts, ignite our imagination, and inspire us to rise above adversity. They remind us that within the tapestry of life, there are narratives that unfold beneath the surface, weaving together moments of strength, resilience, and unwavering courage. One such story is that of Fredrick, a man who embraced life's rhythm despite the challenges imposed by Congestive Heart Failure (CHF). His journey, like a mesmerizing melody, illustrates the power of the human spirit to thrive amidst the backdrop of a chronic condition.

Fredrick's story begins as a symphony of vitality, a life filled with boundless energy, enthusiasm, and purpose. He reveled in the joys of his family, the exhilaration of his career, and the wonders of the world around him. Each day, he moved to the rhythm of life, guided by the beat of his heart that pumped life-giving blood throughout his body.

However, as fate would have it, Fredrick's rhythm started to falter. Gradually, a weariness settled in, an uninvited guest that drained his energy and dimmed the sparkle in his eyes. The symptoms of Congestive Heart Failure crept into his existence, casting a shadow on the vibrant life he once knew. It was as if the once-harmonious melody of his existence had been disrupted, replaced by a dissonant cacophony of uncertainty and fear.

Yet, in the face of this formidable challenge, Fredrick chose not to succumb to despair. Instead, he resolved to embrace life courageously, navigating the ebb and flow of his condition with grace and determination. He sought solace in the arms of his loved ones, finding strength in their unwavering support and encouragement. With their love as his compass, he ventured into the uncharted territory of living with CHF, forging a new path illuminated by resilience and hope.

Fredrick's journey taught him the importance of understanding Congestive Heart Failure, its causes, and its impact on his physical and emotional well-being. He delved into the depths of medical knowledge, exploring the stages of the condition and the array of treatment options available. Armed with this knowledge, he made informed decisions, empowering himself to actively participate in his own care.

Beyond the medical aspects, Fredrick recognized the significance of cultivating a courageous mindset. He confronted his fears head-on, refusing to let them dictate his journey. He discovered the transformative power of resilience, bouncing back from setbacks and finding strength in his ability to adapt. Fredrick sought solace in the company of others who shared his experiences, leaning on their wisdom and support to overcome the emotional challenges that often accompanied living with CHF.

Recognizing the impact of lifestyle choices on his heart health, Fredrick embraced a new way of living. He revamped his diet, adopting heart-healthy nutrition that nourished his body and mind. He discovered the benefits of regular exercise, finding joy and empowerment in physical activities that were suitable for his condition. Fredrick also explored stress management techniques, recognizing the importance of finding balance and serenity amidst life's demands.

In his journey with CHF, Fredrick discovered the vital role that medications and medical management played in his well-being. He became familiar with the array of medications commonly prescribed for CHF, understanding their benefits and potential side effects. Regular medical check-ups became a cornerstone of his routine, ensuring that his condition was carefully monitored, and adjustments to his treatment plan were made as needed. Fredrick also gained insights into various medical procedures and surgeries that could potentially improve his quality of life.

As Fredrick continued his voyage, he navigated the intricacies of everyday life with CHF. He learned to adapt to a new normal, finding innovative ways to pursue his passions and fulfill his responsibilities. Balancing work and lifestyle became a delicate dance, as he discovered the importance of pacing himself and prioritizing self-care. Fredrick's thirst for adventure remained undiminished, and he embarked on travels and vacations, armed with knowledge and strategies to manage his condition while making lasting memories.

Deep within the folds of his journey, Fredrick recognized the significance of nurturing relationships and tending to his emotional well-being. He embraced open and honest communication with his loved ones, inviting them into his world and sharing the intricacies of his condition. Fredrick discovered the importance of intimacy and sexual health, engaging in heartfelt conversations with his partner to ensure that their connection remained strong. He acknowledged the emotional challenges that sometimes accompanied living with CHF and sought professional mental health support when needed.

Along his path, Fredrick encountered others who shared his experiences, each with their unique story of courage and resilience. These inspiring individuals became beacons of hope, reminding him that he was not alone in his journey. Their tales of triumph over adversity ignited a fire within him, spurring him onward and encouraging him to celebrate the victories, big and small, that dotted his own path.

As Fredrick looked towards the future, he discovered the promise of ongoing research and advancements in CHF treatment. He remained committed to maintaining his long-term health and wellness, understanding that his actions today would shape the trajectory of his journey tomorrow. Fredrick recognized the importance of advocacy and support, lending his voice to raise awareness about CHF and providing solace to others who were navigating similar waters.

Beneath the Rhythm: Living Courageously with Congestive Heart Failure is an exploration of Fredrick's journey, woven together with the wisdom, insights, and experiences of countless others who have faced the challenges of CHF head-on. Within these pages, you will discover a tapestry of knowledge, inspiration, and practical guidance to support you on your own courageous journey. May the stories shared within empower you to embrace life's rhythm, to face the challenges of CHF with resilience, and to live courageously, finding beauty and strength in each beat of your heart.

Overview of Congestive Heart Failure (CHF)

In the intricate symphony of the human body, the heart takes center stage, tirelessly orchestrating the flow of life. But sometimes, amidst the harmony, a discordant note emerges. This dissonance is known as Congestive Heart Failure (CHF), a condition that affects millions worldwide, altering the lives of those who hear its somber tune.

CHF is not a single entity, but rather a complex syndrome that arises when the heart's ability to pump blood is compromised, leading to a cascade of physiological imbalances. It is a condition that demands attention, understanding, and a resolute commitment to living courageously.

At its core, CHF stems from various underlying causes, each adding its unique strain to the heart's symphony. Coronary artery disease, high blood pressure, heart valve disorders, and weakened heart muscle due to infections or previous heart attacks are among the chief contributors to this condition. As these ailments take their toll, the heart's pumping efficiency diminishes, impeding the circulation of oxygen-rich blood throughout the body.

One of the defining characteristics of CHF is the insidious onset of its symptoms, which can often be mistaken for the wear and tear of daily life. Fatigue, shortness of breath, persistent coughing, swelling in the legs and ankles, and a reduced ability to exercise are some of the telltale signs that the heart's melody is faltering. As CHF progresses, these symptoms intensify, creating a relentless burden that affects both physical well-being and emotional equilibrium.

The impact of CHF extends far beyond the physical realm. The emotional toll of living with a chronic condition can be profound, weaving a tapestry of fear, anxiety, and uncertainty. Simple tasks that were once taken for granted become monumental challenges, as the specter of CHF casts a shadow on every aspect of life. Yet, within the depths of this darkness, there is an opportunity to discover the transformative power of resilience and the unwavering courage to confront adversity head-on.

While CHF poses formidable challenges, it is not an invincible foe. Modern medicine has gifted us with a repertoire of treatment options that can alleviate symptoms, slow disease progression, and improve quality of life. Medications such as ACE inhibitors, beta-blockers, diuretics, and aldosterone antagonists play a vital role in managing CHF, helping to relieve the strain on the heart and restore balance to the body's intricate systems. For some individuals, medical procedures such as coronary artery bypass grafting, heart valve repair or replacement, and implantation of ventricular assist devices or pacemakers may be necessary to restore the heart's rhythm and function.

Beyond medical interventions, lifestyle modifications serve as a powerful instrument in the fight against CHF. Adopting a heart-healthy diet, low in sodium and saturated fats, can significantly reduce the burden on the heart. Regular physical activity, tailored to an individual's capabilities, can strengthen the heart muscle and improve overall cardiovascular health. Managing stress, maintaining a healthy weight, and abstaining from harmful habits such as smoking or excessive alcohol consumption are additional measures that empower individuals to regain control over their lives.

Navigating the tumultuous seas of CHF requires unwavering vigilance and a commitment to ongoing care. Regular monitoring by healthcare professionals, including routine check-ups, diagnostic tests, and adjustments to medication dosages, ensures that treatment remains optimized. Self-care becomes paramount, as individuals learn to recognize the signs and symptoms of worsening CHF, allowing for early intervention and prevention of exacerbations.

While CHF is an unwelcome companion, it is not a sentence to a life devoid of purpose or joy. With the right tools, knowledge, and support, individuals can reclaim their lives, forging a path that transcends the limitations imposed by their condition. Living courageously with CHF demands resilience, a willingness to adapt, and a steadfast determination to seize each moment with an unwavering spirit.

As we delve deeper into the realm of living courageously with CHF in the pages that follow, let us remember that CHF is not the final note of our symphony. Rather, it is an invitation to create a melody of strength, hope, and resilience, crafting a harmonious existence beneath the rhythm of life.

Purpose of the Book

The purpose of "Beneath the Rhythm: Living Courageously with Congestive Heart Failure" is to serve as a guiding light, a source of knowledge, inspiration, and practical guidance for individuals living with CHF and their loved ones. It is a beacon of hope in the face of adversity, offering solace and encouragement to those navigating the challenging terrain of this chronic condition.

This book aims to provide a comprehensive understanding of CHF, from its causes and symptoms to its impact on physical and emotional well-being. By delving into the intricacies of the condition, it empowers individuals with the knowledge they need to actively participate in their own care, make informed decisions, and effectively communicate with their healthcare team.

Moreover, "Beneath the Rhythm" seeks to foster a courageous mindset in those living with CHF. It encourages individuals to embrace life's challenges head-on, confront their fears, and cultivate resilience in the face of adversity. Through stories of real-life individuals who have found strength and courage in their own CHF journeys, this book serves as a testament to the indomitable human spirit and the power to thrive, even in the face of chronic illness.

The book also recognizes the crucial role of lifestyle modifications in managing CHF. It provides practical guidance on adopting heart-healthy habits, such as nutrition, exercise, stress management, and self-care, to improve overall well-being and enhance quality of life.

Furthermore, "Beneath the Rhythm" acknowledges the importance of relationships and emotional well-being in the CHF journey. It explores strategies for effective communication with loved ones, addresses intimacy and sexual health concerns, and offers guidance on coping with the emotional challenges that often accompany living with CHF. Additionally, it emphasizes the significance of seeking professional mental health support when needed.

As a comprehensive resource, this book delves into medical management options, including medications, medical procedures, and surgeries commonly used to treat CHF. It highlights the importance of regular medical check-ups, monitoring, and compliance with treatment plans to optimize health outcomes.

"Beneath the Rhythm" also celebrates stories of courage and resilience from individuals who have triumphed over the challenges of CHF. By sharing these inspiring narratives, it aims to uplift and motivate readers, reminding them that they are not alone in their journey and that there is hope, even in the face of adversity.

Lastly, this book looks towards the future, discussing promising research and advancements in CHF treatment. It emphasizes the importance of maintaining long-term health and wellness, advocating for CHF awareness, and supporting individuals in embracing a life that transcends the limitations imposed by their condition.

Ultimately, the purpose of "Beneath the Rhythm: Living Courageously with Congestive Heart Failure" is to provide a comprehensive guide, a source of empowerment, and a wellspring of hope for individuals with CHF. It aspires to be a companion on their journey, equipping them with the knowledge, inspiration, and practical tools needed to navigate the challenges of CHF and live a life filled with resilience, courage, and unwavering determination.

Understanding Congestive Heart Failure

Congestive Heart Failure (CHF) is a chronic condition that occurs when the heart's ability to pump blood is compromised, resulting in a cascade of symptoms and physiological imbalances. It is a complex syndrome that requires careful management and ongoing medical care.

To understand CHF, it's important to grasp the basics of how the heart functions. The heart is a muscular organ responsible for pumping oxygen-rich blood to the body's tissues and organs. It has four chambers: two atria and two ventricles. The right side of the heart receives oxygen-depleted blood from the body and pumps it to the lungs to pick up oxygen. The oxygenated blood then returns to the left side of the heart, which pumps it out to the rest of the body.

In CHF, the heart's pumping efficiency becomes impaired, leading to a backlog of blood in the heart and a decrease in the amount of blood being circulated throughout the body. This inadequate blood flow can cause a variety of symptoms and complications.

There are two main types of CHF: systolic heart failure and diastolic heart failure. Systolic heart failure occurs when the heart muscle weakens and fails to contract effectively, leading to reduced pumping ability. Diastolic heart failure, on the other hand, happens when the heart muscle becomes stiff and loses its ability to relax and fill with blood properly.

Various factors can contribute to the development of CHF. Coronary artery disease, which occurs when the blood vessels that supply the heart become narrowed or blocked, is one of the leading causes. High blood pressure, heart valve disorders, previous heart attacks, infections, and certain congenital heart defects can also contribute to the development of CHF.

The symptoms of CHF can vary depending on the severity of the condition. Common signs and symptoms include:

Fatigue and weakness: Reduced blood flow to the muscles and organs can lead to feelings of exhaustion and decreased energy levels.

Shortness of breath: Fluid buildup in the lungs can result in difficulty breathing, especially during physical exertion or when lying flat.

Swelling: Fluid retention may cause swelling in the legs, ankles, feet, or abdomen.

Persistent cough: Fluid accumulation in the lungs can cause a chronic cough that may be accompanied by frothy or pink-tinged sputum.

Rapid or irregular heartbeat: The heart may struggle to maintain a regular rhythm, leading to palpitations or a sensation of a racing or pounding heart.

Reduced exercise tolerance: Due to decreased pumping ability, individuals with CHF may experience difficulty engaging in physical activities they once enjoyed.

If you experience any of these symptoms, it is crucial to consult a healthcare professional for a proper diagnosis and appropriate management.

The management of CHF focuses on relieving symptoms, slowing disease progression, and improving quality of life. Treatment strategies often include medications such as ACE inhibitors, beta-blockers, diuretics, and aldosterone antagonists, which help reduce the workload on the heart, remove excess fluid, and improve cardiac function.

Lifestyle modifications are also an essential component of CHF management. These can include adopting a heart-healthy diet low in sodium and saturated fats, engaging in regular physical activity as tolerated, managing stress levels, maintaining a healthy weight, and abstaining from smoking or excessive alcohol consumption.

In severe cases of CHF that do not respond to medications and lifestyle changes, medical procedures or surgeries may be considered. These can include coronary artery bypass grafting, heart valve repair or replacement, implantation of ventricular assist devices, or heart transplantation.

Regular follow-up appointments with healthcare professionals, including cardiologists and other specialists, are important for monitoring the condition, adjusting medications as needed, and addressing any new symptoms or concerns.

Overall, understanding CHF involves recognizing its underlying causes, identifying its symptoms, and actively managing the condition through a combination of medical interventions, lifestyle modifications, and ongoing care. With proper management and support, individuals with CHF can lead fulfilling lives, maintaining their overall well-being and quality of life.

Definition and Causes

Congestive Heart Failure (CHF) is a chronic condition characterized by the heart's inability to pump blood efficiently, leading to a reduced supply of oxygen and nutrients to the body's tissues and organs. It is often referred to as "heart failure," although it does not mean the heart has completely stopped working.

The causes of CHF can vary and may include:

Coronary Artery Disease (CAD): CAD is the most common cause of CHF. It occurs when the blood vessels that supply oxygen and nutrients to the heart become narrowed or blocked due to the buildup of plaque, restricting blood flow.

High Blood Pressure (Hypertension): Uncontrolled high blood pressure can strain the heart over time, causing it to weaken and become less effective at pumping blood.

Heart Attack: A heart attack, also known as a myocardial infarction, occurs when there is a sudden blockage in the blood flow to a part of the heart muscle. This can cause damage to the heart and impair its pumping ability.

Heart Valve Disorders: Conditions such as mitral valve regurgitation or aortic stenosis, which involve problems with the heart valves, can lead to CHF by affecting the heart's ability to pump blood effectively.

Cardiomyopathy: Cardiomyopathy is a disease of the heart muscle, where the muscle becomes weakened, enlarged, or stiff. This can interfere with the heart's ability to pump blood efficiently and contribute to CHF.

Congenital Heart Defects: Some individuals may be born with structural abnormalities in their heart, such as septal defects (holes in the heart) or valve malformations. These defects can affect normal heart function and potentially lead to CHF later in life.

Arrhythmias: Abnormal heart rhythms, such as atrial fibrillation or ventricular tachycardia, can disrupt the heart's pumping action and contribute to the development of CHF.

Other Factors: Certain factors can increase the risk of developing CHF or worsen existing heart failure, including obesity, diabetes, thyroid disorders, kidney disease, lung disease, excessive alcohol consumption, and drug abuse.

It's important to note that in some cases, the exact cause of CHF may not be identified, and it may result from a combination of factors.

Understanding the underlying causes of CHF is crucial for appropriate diagnosis, treatment, and management. Healthcare professionals evaluate an individual's medical history, perform physical examinations, and conduct various diagnostic tests, such as echocardiograms, electrocardiograms (ECGs), stress tests, and blood tests, to determine the cause and severity of CHF.

Effective management of CHF involves addressing the underlying causes, managing symptoms, and minimizing further damage to the heart. Treatment may include medications to improve heart function, control blood pressure, and reduce fluid retention. Lifestyle modifications, such as adopting a heart-healthy diet, engaging in regular physical activity, quitting smoking, and limiting alcohol intake, can also play a vital role in managing CHF.

In some cases, medical procedures or surgeries may be recommended, such as coronary artery bypass grafting, valve repair or replacement, implantation of medical devices (pacemakers, defibrillators), or, in severe cases, heart transplantation.

It's important for individuals with CHF to work closely with their healthcare team to develop an individualized treatment plan and receive regular monitoring and support to manage their condition effectively.

Symptoms and Diagnosis

Symptoms of Congestive Heart Failure (CHF) can vary depending on the severity of the condition and the specific underlying causes. It's important to note that individuals may not experience all of these symptoms, and the presence of these symptoms does not necessarily indicate CHF. Some common symptoms of CHF include:

Fatigue and Weakness: Feeling constantly tired or lacking energy, even after restful sleep or minimal physical exertion.

Shortness of Breath (Dyspnea): Difficulty breathing, especially during physical activity or when lying flat. Some individuals may also experience sudden shortness of breath during sleep, waking up gasping for air.

Persistent Cough: A chronic cough that may produce white or pink-tinged phlegm. This cough may worsen when lying down or during physical activity.

Fluid Retention and Swelling (Edema): Accumulation of fluid in the legs, ankles, feet, or abdomen. This can cause swelling, tightness, or discomfort in these areas.

Rapid or Irregular Heartbeat: Palpitations or a sensation of a racing or irregular heartbeat.

Reduced Exercise Tolerance: Inability to engage in physical activities or exercise at the same intensity or duration as before due to breathlessness or fatigue.

Weight Gain: Unexplained weight gain or rapid fluctuations in weight due to fluid retention.

Lack of Appetite and Nausea: Loss of appetite, feelings of fullness, or nausea, which can be associated with fluid buildup in the abdomen.

Diagnosis of CHF involves a comprehensive evaluation by a healthcare professional. The diagnostic process may include:

Medical History: The healthcare provider will inquire about your symptoms, medical history, family history of heart disease, and any risk factors or conditions that may contribute to CHF.

Physical Examination: A thorough physical examination will be conducted to assess for signs of fluid retention, abnormal heart sounds, irregular heart rhythms, and other indicators of heart failure.

Diagnostic Tests: Several tests may be ordered to confirm the diagnosis and assess the severity of CHF. These tests may include:

Echocardiogram: This ultrasound test provides detailed images of the heart's structure and function, allowing the healthcare provider to evaluate the heart's pumping ability, valve function, and detect any structural abnormalities.

Electrocardiogram (ECG): This test records the electrical activity of the heart, helping to identify any abnormal rhythms or patterns.

Chest X-ray: X-ray images of the chest can reveal if the heart is enlarged, if there is fluid accumulation in the lungs, or other abnormalities.

Blood Tests: Blood samples can be analyzed to assess kidney function, check for certain markers of heart failure, and rule out other possible causes of symptoms.

Stress Test: This test measures how the heart responds to physical exertion, usually on a treadmill or stationary bike. It helps evaluate the heart's performance under stress and detect any abnormalities.

Cardiac Catheterization: In some cases, a cardiac catheterization may be performed to assess the blood flow in the coronary arteries and evaluate the heart's overall function.

Additional Tests: Depending on the specific circumstances, additional tests such as nuclear imaging, cardiac MRI, or pulmonary function tests may be ordered to gather more detailed information about the heart and lungs.

It's important to consult with a healthcare professional if you experience any symptoms that may suggest CHF. Early diagnosis and treatment can help manage symptoms, slow disease progression, and improve quality of life. Healthcare professionals will develop an individualized treatment plan based on the specific needs and underlying causes of each individual's CHF.

Stages of CHF

Congestive Heart Failure (CHF) is often categorized into different stages based on the severity and progression of the condition. These stages help healthcare professionals assess the extent of heart failure, determine appropriate treatment strategies, and monitor the progression of the disease. The stages of CHF are commonly classified using the New York Heart Association (NYHA) functional classification or the American College of Cardiology/American Heart Association (ACC/AHA) staging system.

Here are the stages of CHF according to the ACC/AHA staging system:

Stage A: At this stage, individuals are at high risk of developing CHF but do not have any structural heart problems or symptoms. This stage typically includes individuals with risk factors such as hypertension, diabetes, coronary artery disease, obesity, or a family history of heart failure. The focus is on managing and treating these risk factors to prevent the development of CHF.

Stage B: In stage B, individuals have structural heart abnormalities, such as a previous heart attack, valve disease, or an enlarged heart, but do not experience symptoms of heart failure. Treatment aims to manage the underlying heart conditions, prevent further damage, and reduce the risk of developing symptomatic heart failure.

Stage C: This stage represents symptomatic heart failure, where individuals have experienced symptoms such as fatigue, shortness of breath, or fluid retention. At this stage, individuals may have reduced exercise tolerance and may experience symptoms even at rest. Treatment focuses on managing symptoms, improving quality of life, and reducing hospitalizations. Medications such as diuretics, ACE inhibitors, beta-blockers, and other medications may be prescribed to improve heart function and relieve symptoms.

Stage D: Stage D represents advanced heart failure, where individuals have severe symptoms and have difficulty carrying out daily activities. Despite optimal medical therapy, they may experience recurrent hospitalizations or require specialized interventions such as cardiac resynchronization therapy, implantable cardioverter-defibrillators (ICDs), or heart transplantation. Palliative care and end-of-life considerations may also be part of the treatment plan at this stage.

It's important to note that the classification of stages may vary based on the specific guidelines or classifications used by healthcare professionals or organizations. The stages provide a general framework for understanding the progression of CHF, but individual cases can vary, and healthcare professionals consider various factors when determining an individual's stage and appropriate treatment options.

Regular follow-up appointments with healthcare professionals are crucial for monitoring the progression of CHF and adjusting treatment plans as needed. By effectively managing CHF at each stage, individuals can optimize their quality of life, minimize symptoms, and slow the progression of the disease.

Treatment Options

The treatment options for Congestive Heart Failure (CHF) aim to alleviate symptoms, slow disease progression, improve heart function, and enhance overall quality of life. The specific treatment plan will depend on the severity of CHF, underlying causes, individual patient characteristics, and the stage of heart failure. It is important to note that treatment for CHF is typically a combination of lifestyle modifications, medications, and, in some cases, surgical interventions. Here are some common treatment options:

Lifestyle Modifications:
Dietary Changes: A heart-healthy diet low in sodium (salt), saturated fats, and cholesterol is recommended. This may include consuming fruits, vegetables,

whole grains, lean proteins, and limiting processed foods.

Fluid Restriction: In advanced stages of CHF, fluid intake may need to be monitored and restricted to prevent fluid overload.

Regular Physical Activity: Exercise, as recommended by the healthcare professional, can help improve heart function, increase stamina, and enhance overall well-being. Individualized exercise programs are designed to meet the patient's abilities and limitations.

Smoking Cessation: Quitting smoking is crucial, as smoking damages blood vessels, increases blood pressure, and exacerbates heart failure symptoms.

Weight Management: Achieving and maintaining a healthy weight can reduce the strain on the heart and improve overall cardiovascular health.

Medications:

Diuretics: Diuretics help eliminate excess fluid from the body, reducing symptoms of fluid retention such as swelling and shortness of breath.

ACE Inhibitors (Angiotensin-Converting Enzyme Inhibitors) and ARBs (Angiotensin Receptor Blockers): These medications help dilate blood vessels, lower blood pressure, and reduce the workload on the heart.

Beta-Blockers: Beta-blockers slow the heart rate, decrease blood pressure, and improve heart function.

Aldosterone Antagonists: These medications help reduce fluid retention and minimize the effects of certain hormones that contribute to heart failure.

Digitalis: Digitalis medications may be prescribed in some cases to strengthen the heart's contractions.

Other Medications: Depending on the specific needs and underlying causes of CHF, additional medications may be prescribed, such as vasodilators, inotropic agents, or anticoagulants to prevent blood clots.

Surgical and Interventional Procedures:

Coronary Artery Bypass Grafting (CABG): In cases where CHF is caused by severe blockages in the coronary arteries, CABG may be performed to improve blood flow to the heart.

Heart Valve Repair or Replacement: If faulty heart valves contribute to CHF, surgical procedures may be performed to repair or replace the affected valves.

Cardiac Resynchronization Therapy (CRT): CRT involves the implantation of a device that coordinates the contractions of the heart's chambers, improving its pumping efficiency.

Implantable Cardioverter-Defibrillator (ICD): ICDs are implanted to monitor heart rhythms and deliver electrical shocks if life-threatening arrhythmias occur.

Ventricular Assist Devices (VADs): VADs are mechanical pumps implanted in individuals with severe heart failure to help the heart pump blood more effectively. They can be used as a bridge to heart transplantation or as destination therapy for individuals who are not eligible for transplantation.

Heart Transplantation: In advanced stages of CHF, heart transplantation may be considered for eligible candidates with end-stage heart failure.

Cardiac Rehabilitation:

Cardiac rehabilitation programs offer comprehensive support, including exercise training, education, and counseling, to help individuals with CHF regain physical strength, manage symptoms, and improve their overall quality of life.

The treatment plan for CHF is individualized, and close collaboration between the patient and the healthcare team is crucial. Regular follow-up appointments are necessary to monitor the effectiveness of treatment, adjust medications, address any complications, and provide ongoing support for self-care management. It is important for individuals with CHF to adhere to their treatment plan, make necessary lifestyle modifications, and communicate any changes in symptoms

to their healthcare provider promptly.

Embracing a Courageous Mindset

Embracing a courageous mindset is an essential component of living with Congestive Heart Failure (CHF) and facing the challenges it presents. While CHF can be a daunting condition, adopting a courageous mindset empowers individuals to navigate their journey with strength, resilience, and determination. Here are key aspects of embracing a courageous mindset when living with CHF:

Acceptance: Accepting the diagnosis of CHF and its impact on daily life is the first step towards embracing courage. Acknowledge the reality of the condition, understand its challenges, and recognize that it is a part of your life. Acceptance allows you to move forward and focus on proactive steps towards managing the condition effectively.

Positive Attitude: Cultivating a positive mindset is essential. Choose to focus on what you can control rather than dwelling on limitations or setbacks. Positivity fuels resilience, inspires hope, and helps overcome obstacles. Surround yourself with a support system of loved ones, healthcare professionals, and fellow CHF warriors who uplift and encourage you on your journey.

Education and Empowerment: Take an active role in learning about CHF. Educate yourself about the condition, its symptoms, treatment options, and self-care strategies. Knowledge empowers you to make informed decisions, communicate effectively with your healthcare team, and actively participate in your own care. Stay updated on the latest research and developments in CHF management.

Self-Care and Lifestyle Modifications: Prioritize self-care and adopt healthy lifestyle habits that support your overall well-being. Follow your healthcare team's recommendations regarding medications, diet, exercise, stress management, and adequate rest. Engaging in self-care activities such as relaxation techniques, hobbies, and pursuing interests outside of CHF can help maintain a positive mindset and enhance quality of life.

Courageous Communication: Open and honest communication with your healthcare team and loved ones is crucial. Share your concerns, ask questions, and seek clarification about your condition and treatment plan. Effective communication ensures that you receive the support and information you need to manage CHF effectively.

Gratitude and Mindfulness: Cultivate a sense of gratitude for the things that bring joy, meaning, and purpose to your life. Practice mindfulness by being fully present in each moment and appreciating the small victories and blessings. Gratitude and mindfulness can help reduce stress, promote emotional well-being, and enhance overall resilience.

Celebrate Progress: Recognize and celebrate your progress, no matter how small. Overcoming challenges and taking steps towards managing CHF is an achievement worthy of celebration. Embrace a growth mindset and focus on the progress you have made rather than dwelling on setbacks.

Support Networks: Seek out and engage with support networks and CHF communities. Connecting with others who share similar experiences can provide invaluable emotional support, understanding, and practical tips for managing CHF. Online forums, support groups, and advocacy organizations can serve as sources of inspiration, encouragement, and knowledge-sharing.

Remember, embracing a courageous mindset is not about denying the difficulties of CHF but rather acknowledging them and choosing to face them with determination, resilience, and a positive outlook. By embracing a courageous mindset, you can live each day to the fullest, finding strength within yourself to overcome challenges and create a meaningful life despite CHF.

Facing Fear and Overcoming Challenges

Facing fear and overcoming challenges are integral aspects of living courageously with Congestive Heart Failure (CHF). While it is natural to feel fear and encounter obstacles along the way, adopting strategies to confront and transcend these challenges can empower individuals with CHF to lead fulfilling lives. Here are some approaches to facing fear and overcoming challenges:

Acknowledge and Understand Fear: Recognize that fear is a normal response when facing a chronic health condition like CHF. Take the time to understand what specifically triggers your fears and anxieties. By identifying the root causes, you can develop strategies to address and mitigate them effectively.

Seek Support: Reach out to your support network, including family, friends, healthcare professionals, or support groups. Sharing your fears and concerns with others who understand and empathize can provide comfort, encouragement, and practical advice. Sometimes, simply expressing your feelings can help alleviate fear and make challenges seem more manageable.

Educate Yourself: Knowledge is power. Educate yourself about CHF, its treatment options, and strategies for managing symptoms. The more you understand your condition, the better equipped you will be to make informed decisions and overcome challenges. Ask your healthcare team for educational resources or reputable websites where you can learn more.

Develop Coping Strategies: Explore various coping mechanisms to manage fear and stress. These may include relaxation techniques (such as deep breathing exercises or meditation), journaling, engaging in hobbies or activities that bring you joy, or seeking professional counseling or therapy. Find what works best for you and integrate it into your daily routine.

Set Realistic Goals: Break down your challenges into smaller, achievable goals. This approach allows you to focus on one step at a time, creating a sense of progress and accomplishment. Celebrate each milestone, no matter how small, as it demonstrates your resilience and ability to overcome adversity.

Practice Self-Compassion: Be kind to yourself during challenging times. Understand that setbacks and difficulties are part of the journey. Treat yourself with compassion, patience, and self-care. Practice positive self-talk and remind yourself of your strength, resilience, and the progress you have made.

Embrace Mindfulness: Stay present in the moment and cultivate mindfulness. Mindfulness can help alleviate anxiety and fear by grounding you in the present reality rather than dwelling on past experiences or worrying about the future. Practice mindfulness techniques such as deep breathing, focusing on your senses, or engaging in activities mindfully.

Seek Professional Guidance: If fear and anxiety become overwhelming, consider seeking professional help from therapists, psychologists, or counselors specializing in chronic illness or anxiety management. They can provide you with tools and strategies tailored to your specific needs to help you navigate your challenges more effectively.

Celebrate Resilience: Take the time to acknowledge and celebrate your resilience. Recognize the strength and courage it takes to face and overcome challenges. Reflect on past experiences where you have triumphed over difficulties, and draw inspiration from those moments as you confront new challenges.

Remember, facing fear and overcoming challenges is a personal journey, and it is okay to ask for help along the way. By adopting a proactive and resilient mindset, you can navigate the challenges of CHF with courage, determination, and a sense of empowerment.

Cultivating Resilience

Cultivating resilience is a powerful mindset and skill that can greatly benefit individuals living with Congestive Heart Failure (CHF). Resilience enables individuals to adapt, cope, and bounce back from the challenges and setbacks that arise due to CHF. Here are some strategies for cultivating resilience:

Develop a Positive Mindset: Cultivate a positive outlook by focusing on strengths, possibilities, and gratitude. Train your mind to see challenges as opportunities for growth and learning rather than insurmountable obstacles. Embrace a belief in your ability to overcome difficulties and find solutions.

Build a Supportive Network: Surround yourself with a strong support system of family, friends, healthcare professionals, and support groups who understand and uplift you. Seek out individuals who provide emotional support, encouragement, and practical assistance. Sharing experiences and receiving support can bolster resilience.

Practice Self-Care: Prioritize self-care to nurture your physical, mental, and emotional well-being. Engage in activities that bring you joy, relaxation, and fulfillment. This may include exercise, meditation, hobbies, spending time in nature, or engaging in creative outlets. Taking care of yourself empowers you to face challenges with renewed energy and resilience.

Foster Effective Coping Mechanisms: Develop healthy coping strategies to manage stress, anxiety, and emotional difficulties. This may involve deep breathing exercises, journaling, practicing mindfulness or relaxation techniques, seeking therapy or counseling, or engaging in activities that promote stress relief. Find coping mechanisms that resonate with you and incorporate them into your daily routine.

Set Realistic Goals: Set achievable goals and break them down into smaller, manageable steps. This approach allows you to make progress and experience a sense of accomplishment along the way. Celebrate your achievements, no matter how small, as they contribute to building resilience and confidence.

Maintain Open Communication: Effective communication with your healthcare team, loved ones, and support network is vital. Express your needs, concerns, and fears openly. Seek clarification, ask questions, and engage in collaborative decision-making about your treatment plan. Effective communication fosters understanding, support, and empowerment.

Adaptability and Flexibility: Cultivate adaptability and flexibility in the face of changing circumstances and setbacks. Recognize that adjustments may be necessary along your journey with CHF. Embrace the ability to adapt your goals, treatment plan, and self-care strategies as needed. Flexibility allows you to navigate challenges with resilience and find new pathways forward.

Embrace Education: Continuously educate yourself about CHF, advancements in treatments, self-care strategies, and new research. Knowledge empowers you to make informed decisions, actively participate in your care, and advocate for yourself. Seek reputable sources of information, attend educational workshops, and stay engaged in your healthcare journey.

Practice Mindfulness and Acceptance: Embrace mindfulness and practice acceptance of your current situation. Mindfulness helps you stay present in the moment, fostering resilience by reducing stress and anxiety. Acceptance allows you to acknowledge the realities of CHF while focusing on proactive steps to manage and adapt to the condition.

Cultivate a Sense of Purpose: Find meaning and purpose in your life beyond CHF. Engage in activities, hobbies, or pursuits that bring you fulfillment, joy, and a sense of purpose. Connecting with a greater purpose can provide motivation, resilience, and a positive outlook.

Remember, resilience is a journey, and it takes time and practice to cultivate. Embrace each day with a resilient mindset, drawing on your strengths and support systems as you navigate the challenges of CHF. With resilience, you can face adversity head-on and lead a fulfilling and meaningful life despite the condition.

Seeking support: friends, family, and community

Seeking support from friends, family, and the community is an invaluable resource for individuals living with Congestive Heart Failure (CHF). The journey of managing CHF can be challenging, both physically and emotionally, and having a strong support system can provide comfort, encouragement, and practical assistance. Here are some ways to seek support from your loved ones and community:

Open Communication: Foster open and honest communication with your friends and family members. Share your experiences, concerns, and needs with them. Let them know how CHF impacts your life and how they can support you.

Encourage them to ask questions and educate themselves about CHF to better understand your condition.

Emotional Support: Seek emotional support from your loved ones. Share your feelings, fears, and anxieties with them. Sometimes, simply having someone to listen to you can provide immense comfort and relief. Expressing your emotions can help you process your experiences and reduce feelings of isolation.

Practical Assistance: Don't hesitate to ask for practical help when you need it. CHF may affect your energy levels, physical abilities, or require lifestyle adjustments. Allow your friends and family to lend a hand with tasks such as grocery shopping, meal preparation, house chores, or transportation to medical appointments. Accepting support can lighten your load and allow you to focus on self-care and managing your condition.

Join Support Groups: Consider joining support groups specifically tailored for individuals living with CHF. These groups provide a safe and understanding environment where you can connect with others who share similar experiences. Sharing stories, tips, and insights with fellow CHF warriors can be empowering, inspiring, and help you feel less alone in your journey.

Online Communities: Explore online communities and forums dedicated to CHF. These platforms allow you to connect with individuals from around the world, sharing knowledge, experiences, and emotional support. Engage in discussions, ask questions, and offer your support to others. Online communities can be accessible resources, particularly for individuals with limited local support options.

Education and Awareness: Encourage your friends, family, and community to educate themselves about CHF. Share educational resources, articles, or websites to help them understand the condition better. Consider organizing awareness events or participating in CHF-related fundraising activities to increase awareness and support within your community.

Caregiver Support: If you have caregivers involved in your CHF management, ensure they receive the necessary support and resources as well. Caregivers play a crucial role in providing assistance and emotional support. Encourage them to join caregiver support groups or seek counseling to address their own needs and challenges.

Community Resources: Research local community resources and organizations that provide support for individuals living with CHF. These may include cardiac rehabilitation programs, counseling services, educational workshops, or community events focused on heart health. Engaging with these resources can expand your support network and provide additional avenues for assistance and guidance.

Remember, seeking support is not a sign of weakness, but rather a recognition of the strength and resilience it takes to face the challenges of CHF. By reaching out to friends, family, and the community, you can create a network of support that empowers you to navigate the ups and downs of living with CHF and enhance your overall well-being.

Living with Hope and Positivity

Living with hope and positivity is a powerful mindset that can greatly impact the experience of living with Congestive Heart Failure (CHF). While CHF presents its challenges, maintaining a hopeful and positive outlook can provide strength, resilience, and improve overall well-being. Here are some strategies for living with hope and positivity:

Focus on the Present: Instead of dwelling on the uncertainties of the future or the difficulties of the past, practice mindfulness and focus on the present moment. Embrace the opportunities and joys that each day brings. Cultivate gratitude for the small blessings in life, such as spending time with loved ones, enjoying nature, or engaging in activities that bring you joy.

Set Realistic Goals: Establish realistic goals that align with your abilities and circumstances. Break them down into manageable steps and celebrate each milestone along the way. By achieving these goals, you'll build confidence and a sense of accomplishment, fostering a positive outlook and hope for the future.

Practice Self-Care: Prioritize self-care to nurture your physical, mental, and emotional well-being. Engage in activities that bring you joy and relaxation, such as exercise, hobbies, or pursuing interests outside of CHF. Take time for rest and relaxation, ensuring you are giving yourself the care and attention you need to thrive.

Surround Yourself with Positivity: Surround yourself with positive influences, including supportive friends, family members, and healthcare professionals who uplift and encourage you. Minimize exposure to negativity and seek out inspirational stories, books, or podcasts that promote hope and resilience. Fill your environment with uplifting and motivating elements that remind you of the possibilities that lie ahead.

Seek Inspiration: Look for role models and individuals who have overcome challenges and thrived despite their health conditions. Their stories can provide inspiration and serve as reminders that it is possible to live a fulfilling life with CHF. Seek out support groups or online communities where you can connect with others who share similar experiences and find inspiration in their journeys.

Practice Positive Self-Talk: Pay attention to your inner dialogue and challenge negative thoughts or self-limiting beliefs. Replace self-doubt and criticism with positive affirmations and encouraging self-talk. Remind yourself of your strengths, resilience, and the progress you have made.

Surround yourself with positive affirmations or create a gratitude journal to reinforce a positive mindset.

Embrace Support Systems: Lean on your support systems, including friends, family, healthcare professionals, and support groups. Share your experiences, concerns, and achievements with them. Seek their guidance, encouragement, and reassurance during challenging times. Engaging with supportive individuals can bolster your sense of hope and provide valuable emotional support.

Engage in Meaningful Activities: Find activities or causes that give you a sense of purpose and fulfillment. Engaging in activities that align with your values and passions can provide a sense of meaning and ignite a sense of hope. This may include volunteering, participating in advocacy work, or pursuing hobbies or creative outlets that bring you joy.

Stay Informed and Empowered: Stay informed about advancements in CHF research, treatment options, and self-care strategies. Knowledge empowers you to make informed decisions about your health and engage actively in your care. Stay connected with your healthcare team and ask questions to ensure you have the information you need to make confident choices.

Cultivate Resilience: Embrace challenges as opportunities for growth and resilience-building. Learn from setbacks, adapt to changes, and view obstacles as temporary roadblocks rather than insurmountable barriers. Cultivating resilience allows you to face challenges with hope, determination, and a belief in your ability to overcome them.

Living with hope and positivity does not mean ignoring the realities of CHF but rather choosing to focus on the possibilities, strengths, and the potential for a fulfilling life. By cultivating a hopeful and positive mindset, you can navigate the challenges of CHF with resilience, optimism, and an unwavering belief in the possibilities that lie ahead.

Lifestyle Changes for Heart Health

Lifestyle changes play a crucial role in promoting heart health and managing conditions like Congestive Heart Failure (CHF). Adopting a heart-healthy lifestyle can improve your overall well-being, reduce symptoms, and enhance your quality of life. Here are some key lifestyle changes that can positively impact heart health:

Healthy Diet: Adopt a balanced and nutritious diet that includes plenty of fruits, vegetables, whole grains, lean proteins, and healthy fats. Limit your intake of saturated and trans fats, cholesterol, sodium, and added sugars. Consider working with a registered dietitian to develop a personalized meal plan that suits your specific dietary needs and restrictions.

Regular Exercise: Engage in regular physical activity as recommended by your healthcare team. Exercise helps improve cardiovascular fitness, strengthen the heart and blood vessels, and manage weight. Choose activities you enjoy and aim for at least 150 minutes of moderate-intensity aerobic exercise or 75 minutes of vigorous-intensity exercise per week. Consult your healthcare provider before starting any new exercise program.

Weight Management: Maintain a healthy weight to reduce the strain on your heart. If overweight, aim for gradual and sustainable weight loss through a combination of a healthy diet and regular physical activity. Your healthcare team can provide guidance on setting realistic weight loss goals and monitoring your progress.

Smoking Cessation: Quit smoking and avoid exposure to secondhand smoke. Smoking damages blood vessels, raises blood pressure, and increases the risk of heart disease. Quitting smoking has immediate and long-term benefits for heart health. Seek support from healthcare professionals, counseling services, or smoking cessation programs to help you quit successfully.

Limit Alcohol Intake: Limit your alcohol consumption to moderate levels. Excessive alcohol intake can contribute to high blood pressure and increase the risk of heart problems. Men should limit themselves to no more than two standard drinks per day, while women should aim for no more than one standard drink per day.

Stress Management: Develop effective stress management techniques to reduce the impact of stress on your heart. Stress can contribute to elevated blood pressure and heart rate. Explore relaxation techniques, such as deep breathing exercises, meditation, yoga, or engaging in activities that promote relaxation and self-care.

Medication Adherence: Take prescribed medications as directed by your healthcare provider. Medications for CHF, such as diuretics, beta-blockers, ACE inhibitors, or angiotensin receptor blockers, help manage symptoms and improve heart function. Follow your medication regimen diligently and discuss any concerns or side effects with your healthcare team.

Regular Medical Check-ups: Attend regular check-ups with your healthcare provider to monitor your heart health and manage CHF effectively. These appointments allow your healthcare team to assess your condition, adjust medications if needed, and provide guidance on lifestyle modifications.

Sleep Quality: Prioritize getting adequate sleep and maintain a consistent sleep schedule. Poor sleep can contribute to high blood pressure and increase the risk of heart problems. Aim for 7-8 hours of quality sleep each night and create a relaxing bedtime routine.

Social Support: Seek and maintain a strong support network of family, friends, and healthcare professionals. Emotional support can play a significant role in managing heart health and coping with the challenges of CHF. Engage in social activities, join support groups, or seek counseling if needed.

Remember, lifestyle changes take time and consistency to yield significant results. It's essential to work closely with your healthcare team to create a personalized plan that suits your specific needs and abilities. By making these positive lifestyle changes, you can optimize heart health, manage CHF effectively, and enhance your overall well-being.

Importance of Diet and Nutrition

Diet and nutrition play a critical role in maintaining good health and preventing various diseases, including cardiovascular conditions like Congestive Heart Failure (CHF). A well-balanced and nutritious diet can support heart health, manage risk factors, and improve overall well-being. Here are some key reasons highlighting the importance of diet and nutrition:

Heart Disease Prevention: A healthy diet is one of the most effective ways to prevent heart disease, including CHF. A diet rich in fruits, vegetables, whole grains, lean proteins, and healthy fats can help control blood pressure, reduce cholesterol levels, prevent the buildup of plaque in the arteries, and promote overall heart health.

Blood Pressure Management: A diet low in sodium and high in potassium, calcium, and magnesium can help manage blood pressure levels. Excess sodium intake can contribute to high blood pressure, which is a significant risk factor for heart disease. Eating a diet rich in fruits, vegetables, whole grains, and low-fat dairy products while limiting processed and packaged foods can help maintain healthy blood pressure levels.

Cholesterol Control: Consuming a diet low in saturated fats and trans fats can help manage cholesterol levels. High levels of LDL (low-density lipoprotein) cholesterol, often referred to as "bad" cholesterol, can increase the risk of heart disease. Incorporating heart-healthy fats, such as those found in avocados, nuts, seeds, and fatty fish, can help increase HDL (high-density lipoprotein) cholesterol, known as "good" cholesterol, and lower LDL cholesterol levels.

Weight Management: A nutritious diet can contribute to maintaining a healthy weight or achieving weight loss, if necessary. Excess weight can strain the heart and increase the risk of heart disease. By consuming a balanced diet that includes appropriate portions and a variety of nutrient-dense foods, you can manage your weight effectively and reduce the burden on your cardiovascular system.

Diabetes Prevention and Management: A well-balanced diet can help prevent and manage diabetes, which is a significant risk factor for heart disease. Consuming foods with a low glycemic index, such as whole grains, legumes, and non-starchy vegetables, can help regulate blood sugar levels. Additionally, choosing foods high in fiber, lean proteins, and healthy fats can promote stable blood sugar control.

Nutrient Supply: A healthy diet provides essential nutrients, vitamins, minerals, and antioxidants that are vital for overall health and proper functioning of the body. Nutrient deficiencies can compromise heart health and increase the risk of various health conditions. Consuming a variety of nutrient-rich foods ensures that your body receives the necessary nutrients to support cardiovascular health.

Energy and Vitality: Proper nutrition is essential for maintaining optimal energy levels and promoting vitality. A well-nourished body is better equipped to handle the demands of daily activities and maintain an active lifestyle. A nutrient-rich diet provides the energy needed for physical activity, which is vital for heart health and overall well-being.

Overall Well-Being: Good nutrition is not only important for physical health but also for mental and emotional well-being. Certain nutrients, such as omega-3 fatty acids, B vitamins, and antioxidants, have been associated with improved mood, cognitive function, and reduced risk of mental health conditions. A healthy diet can positively impact your overall quality of life.

It's important to note that individual dietary needs may vary based on factors such as age, sex, activity level, and underlying health conditions.

Consulting with a registered dietitian or healthcare professional can help you develop a personalized and balanced eating plan that meets your specific needs and supports your heart health goals.

Remember, adopting a healthy diet is a long-term commitment and should be combined with other lifestyle factors such as regular physical activity, stress management, and avoiding tobacco use. By prioritizing diet and nutrition, you can take proactive steps towards promoting heart health, managing CHF, and enjoying a healthier and more fulfilling life.

Managing Fluid Intake

Managing fluid intake is a crucial aspect of self-care for individuals living with Congestive Heart Failure (CHF). CHF can lead to fluid retention in the body, causing symptoms such as swelling, shortness of breath, and fatigue. Proper management of fluid intake helps maintain fluid balance and alleviate symptoms. Here are some strategies for managing fluid intake:

Consult with your healthcare team: It is important to work closely with your healthcare team, including your cardiologist and/or a registered dietitian, to establish fluid intake guidelines that are tailored to your specific condition and needs. They can provide personalized recommendations based on the severity of your CHF, medications, and other individual factors.

Monitor fluid intake: Keep track of your daily fluid intake to ensure you stay within the recommended limits. This includes not only beverages but also foods with high water content, such as soups, fruits, and vegetables. Use measuring cups or containers to accurately measure your fluid intake.

Limit sodium intake: Sodium can contribute to fluid retention. Reduce your sodium intake by avoiding or minimizing processed and packaged foods, as they are often high in sodium. Opt for fresh, whole foods and use herbs and spices to add flavor to your meals instead of salt.

Follow fluid restrictions: In some cases, your healthcare team may recommend specific fluid restrictions. This means you will have a daily limit on the amount of fluid you can consume. Adhere to these restrictions strictly to prevent fluid overload and manage symptoms effectively.

Monitor body weight: Regularly monitor your body weight, preferably on a daily basis, and keep a record of the measurements. Sudden weight gain can be an indicator of fluid retention. Notify your healthcare team if you experience rapid weight gain, as it may require adjustments to your treatment plan.

Understand fluid equivalents: It can be helpful to understand the fluid content of different beverages and foods. For example, a standard serving size of fluids is often considered 8 ounces or 240 milliliters. Be mindful of the fluid content in various beverages and adjust your intake accordingly.

Pace your fluid intake: Instead of consuming large amounts of fluids at once, spread your fluid intake throughout the day. Sipping fluids slowly can help your body better manage fluid balance and reduce the risk of overwhelming your heart and kidneys.

Opt for low-sodium fluids: When choosing beverages, opt for options that are low in sodium. Water is generally the best choice, but you can also consider herbal teas, unsweetened fruit juices (in moderation), and low-sodium broths. Avoid or limit beverages that are high in caffeine or alcohol, as they can have a diuretic effect and contribute to fluid loss.

Be mindful of hidden fluids: Pay attention to hidden sources of fluids in your diet, such as foods with high water content. Soups, fruits, vegetables, and gelatin-based desserts all contain fluids that contribute to your overall intake. Consider these sources when calculating your daily fluid intake.

Communicate with your healthcare team: If you have any concerns, questions, or experience changes in your symptoms, communicate with your healthcare team promptly. They can provide guidance, monitor your progress, and make necessary adjustments to your fluid intake recommendations.

Remember, managing fluid intake is individualized and may vary depending on your specific condition and treatment plan. Work closely with your healthcare team to develop a fluid management strategy that suits your needs and helps optimize your heart health.

Exercise and Physical Activity

Exercise and physical activity play a crucial role in managing Congestive Heart Failure (CHF) and promoting overall heart health. Regular exercise can help improve cardiovascular fitness, strengthen the heart and blood vessels, manage weight, and enhance quality of life. Here are some key points to consider regarding exercise and physical activity for individuals with CHF:

Consult with your healthcare team: Before starting or modifying an exercise program, consult with your healthcare team, including your cardiologist or primary care physician. They can assess your specific condition, provide guidance on exercise intensity and duration, and make recommendations tailored to your needs and abilities.

Aim for a well-rounded exercise routine: Your exercise routine should include a combination of aerobic exercise, strength training, and flexibility exercises. Each component offers unique benefits for heart health and overall fitness.

Aerobic Exercise: Engage in aerobic activities that raise your heart rate and increase breathing, such as brisk walking, cycling, swimming, or low-impact aerobics. Start with shorter durations and gradually increase the time as tolerated. Aim for at least 150 minutes of moderate-intensity aerobic exercise or 75 minutes of vigorous-intensity exercise per week, as recommended by the American Heart Association.

Strength Training: Include strength training exercises that target major muscle groups in your routine. Use resistance bands, dumbbells, or bodyweight exercises to improve muscle strength and endurance. Focus on proper form and start with light weights, gradually increasing the intensity over time. Aim for two or more sessions per week.

Flexibility Exercises: Incorporate stretching and flexibility exercises to maintain joint mobility and prevent muscle tightness. Gentle stretching exercises, yoga, or tai chi can help improve flexibility and balance.

Gradual progression: Start slowly and gradually increase the intensity and duration of your exercise sessions. This allows your body to adapt and minimizes the risk of overexertion or exacerbation of symptoms. Listen to your body and modify your exercise routine as needed.

Pay attention to symptoms: During exercise, be mindful of any symptoms such as chest pain, severe shortness of breath, dizziness, or extreme fatigue. If you experience any of these symptoms, stop exercising and seek medical attention. It's important to differentiate between normal exercise discomfort and symptoms that may require medical intervention.

Monitor heart rate: Monitoring your heart rate during exercise can help you gauge the intensity of your workout. Your healthcare team can provide guidance on your target heart rate range or prescribe a specific heart rate zone for exercise. Use a heart rate monitor or check your pulse manually to ensure you stay within the recommended range.

Stay hydrated: Drink water before, during, and after exercise to maintain proper hydration. Proper hydration supports cardiovascular function and helps regulate body temperature during physical activity.

Listen to your body: Be aware of your body's limitations and adjust your exercise routine accordingly. If you feel fatigued or experience increased shortness of breath, it may be necessary to reduce the intensity or duration of your workout. It's important to find the right balance between pushing yourself and respecting your body's needs.

Be consistent: Consistency is key when it comes to exercise. Aim for regular physical activity and strive to make it a part of your daily routine. Consistency helps maintain cardiovascular fitness, manage weight, and optimize the benefits of exercise.

Consider cardiac rehabilitation: Cardiac rehabilitation programs offer supervised exercise sessions and educational support for individuals with heart conditions, including CHF. These programs are designed to safely guide you through an exercise regimen and provide valuable resources for managing your heart health. Speak to your healthcare team about the availability of cardiac rehabilitation programs in your area.

Enjoy physical activity in daily life: In addition to structured exercise sessions, find ways to incorporate physical activity into your daily life. Take the stairs instead of the elevator, engage in household chores or gardening, or go for leisurely walks. Every bit of activity adds up and contributes to your overall fitness.

Remember, individual exercise recommendations may vary based on the severity of CHF, overall health, and individual circumstances. Work closely with your healthcare team to develop a safe and effective exercise plan that suits your specific needs and abilities. Regular exercise, combined with medical management and other lifestyle modifications, can significantly improve your heart health and overall well-being.

Stress Management and Relaxation Techniques

Stress management and relaxation techniques are essential for individuals living with Congestive Heart Failure (CHF) as they can help reduce the impact of stress on the heart, improve overall well-being, and enhance the effectiveness of medical treatments. Here are some strategies to effectively manage stress and promote relaxation:

Deep Breathing: Practice deep breathing exercises to activate the body's relaxation response. Sit or lie down in a comfortable position, close your eyes, and take slow, deep breaths. Inhale deeply through your nose, allowing your abdomen to rise, and exhale slowly through your mouth, focusing on releasing tension with each breath.

Meditation and Mindfulness: Engage in meditation or mindfulness practices to calm the mind and reduce stress. Find a quiet space, sit in a comfortable position, and focus your attention on your breath, bodily sensations, or a specific calming object. Allow thoughts to come and go without judgment or attachment.

Progressive Muscle Relaxation: This technique involves systematically tensing and relaxing different muscle groups to promote physical and mental relaxation. Start by tensing a specific muscle group, such as your hands, and then release the tension while focusing on the sensation of relaxation. Move through each muscle group, progressively working your way up or down the body.

Guided Imagery: Use guided imagery to create a mental escape and promote relaxation. Close your eyes and visualize a peaceful and calming place, such as a serene beach or a quiet forest. Engage your senses by imagining the sights, sounds, smells, and sensations of this place. Allow yourself to fully immerse in the imagery and experience a sense of relaxation.

Exercise and Physical Activity: Engaging in regular exercise and physical activity not only benefits the body but also helps manage stress and promotes relaxation. Exercise releases endorphins, which are natural mood boosters. Choose activities you enjoy, such as walking, swimming, or yoga, and incorporate them into your routine.

Social Support: Seek support from friends, family, or support groups. Sharing your experiences, concerns, and emotions with others who understand can help alleviate stress and provide a sense of connection. Participating in support groups or talking to a counselor or therapist can also provide valuable guidance and coping strategies.

Time Management: Effective time management can help reduce stress and create a sense of control. Prioritize tasks and responsibilities, delegate when possible, and learn to say no to additional commitments when necessary. Break tasks into smaller, manageable steps and focus on one thing at a time.

Healthy Lifestyle Habits: Adopting healthy lifestyle habits can have a significant impact on stress levels. Maintain a balanced diet, get enough sleep, limit caffeine and alcohol intake, and avoid tobacco and recreational drug use. These lifestyle choices support overall well-being and help manage stress more effectively.

Relaxation Techniques: Explore other relaxation techniques such as aromatherapy, listening to calming music, taking warm baths, or engaging in hobbies that bring you joy and relaxation. Find activities that help you unwind and make time for them regularly.

Professional Help: If stress becomes overwhelming or persists despite self-help efforts, consider seeking professional help. A counselor, therapist, or psychologist can provide guidance and support in developing effective stress management techniques and coping strategies.

Remember, managing stress is a continuous process, and what works for one person may not work for another. Experiment with different techniques and find what resonates with you. By incorporating stress management and relaxation techniques into your daily life, you can better manage stress, enhance your well-being, and support your heart health in living courageously with CHF.

Medication and Medical Management

Medication and medical management are essential components in the treatment and care of individuals living with Congestive Heart Failure (CHF). These interventions aim to alleviate symptoms, improve heart function, prevent disease progression, and enhance overall quality of life. Here are some key aspects of medication and medical management for CHF:

Medication Regimen: Your healthcare team, including your cardiologist and primary care physician, will prescribe medications based on the severity of your CHF, underlying causes, and individual factors. Commonly prescribed medications for CHF include:

Diuretics: Diuretics help reduce fluid retention by increasing urine production and promoting fluid excretion. They alleviate symptoms such as edema (swelling) and shortness of breath.

ACE inhibitors (Angiotensin-Converting Enzyme inhibitors) or ARBs (Angiotensin Receptor Blockers): These medications help relax blood vessels, lower blood pressure, and reduce the workload on the heart.

Beta-Blockers: Beta-blockers slow the heart rate, reduce blood pressure, and improve heart function. They can help control irregular heart rhythms and reduce strain on the heart.

Aldosterone Antagonists: These medications block the effects of the hormone aldosterone, which can contribute to fluid retention and worsen heart failure symptoms.

Digoxin: Digoxin improves heart function and can help control heart rate in certain cases.

Other medications: Depending on your specific condition, additional medications such as vasodilators, anticoagulants, or antiplatelet agents may be prescribed.

It is crucial to take medications exactly as prescribed, follow the recommended dosage, and inform your healthcare team about any side effects or concerns. Regular follow-up appointments will allow your healthcare team to assess the effectiveness of the medications and make adjustments as needed.

Lifestyle Modifications: In addition to medication, your healthcare team will emphasize the importance of lifestyle modifications to manage CHF effectively. This may include:

Dietary changes: A heart-healthy diet low in sodium and saturated fats can help manage CHF. Your healthcare team may recommend a low-sodium diet to control fluid retention and reduce strain on the heart.

Fluid restriction: In some cases, your healthcare team may recommend fluid restrictions to manage fluid overload and symptoms. It is important to adhere to these restrictions and monitor fluid intake carefully.

Regular physical activity: Engaging in regular exercise, as discussed previously, can improve heart function, overall fitness, and quality of life.

Smoking cessation: If you smoke, quitting is crucial to reduce further damage to the heart and blood vessels.

Alcohol moderation: Limiting alcohol intake can help prevent further strain on the heart and reduce the risk of complications.

Weight management: Achieving and maintaining a healthy weight can help improve heart function and reduce symptoms.

Monitoring and Follow-up: Regular monitoring and follow-up appointments are essential to assess your condition, monitor the effectiveness of medications, and make necessary adjustments. Your healthcare team may conduct periodic tests, such as echocardiograms, electrocardiograms (ECGs), or blood tests, to evaluate heart function, check medication levels, and detect any underlying conditions or complications.

Surgical and Interventional Procedures: In some cases, surgical or interventional procedures may be recommended to manage CHF. These procedures can include:

Coronary artery bypass grafting (CABG): It involves bypassing blocked or narrowed coronary arteries to improve blood flow to the heart.

Cardiac resynchronization therapy (CRT): This procedure involves implanting a device to help synchronize the heart's electrical signals and improve its pumping efficiency.

Implantable cardioverter-defibrillator (ICD): An ICD is a device implanted in the chest to monitor and correct potentially life-threatening irregular heart rhythms.

Heart transplantation: In severe cases of CHF, heart transplantation may be considered when other treatments have been ineffective.

Education and Self-care: Education is key to effectively manage CHF. Your healthcare team will provide information about your condition, medications, lifestyle modifications, and warning signs of worsening symptoms. It is important to follow the recommended self-care practices, such as monitoring your weight, recognizing symptoms of fluid retention or worsening heart failure, and seeking prompt medical attention when needed.

Remember, medication and medical management are tailored to each individual's specific condition and may vary. It is crucial to work closely with your healthcare team, ask questions, and actively participate in your care to

optimize the management of CHF and
improve your quality of life.

Common medications of CHF

Several medications are commonly prescribed for the management of Congestive Heart Failure (CHF). Here are some of the main types of medications used in the treatment of CHF:

Diuretics: Diuretics help reduce fluid retention by increasing urine production and promoting the excretion of excess fluid. They are often used to relieve symptoms such as edema (swelling) and shortness of breath. Commonly prescribed diuretics include furosemide (Lasix), hydrochlorothiazide (Microzide), and spironolactone (Aldactone).

Angiotensin-Converting Enzyme (ACE) Inhibitors: ACE inhibitors help relax blood vessels, reduce blood pressure, and decrease the workload on the heart. They can improve symptoms, slow the progression of CHF, and prolong survival. Examples of ACE inhibitors include lisinopril (Prinivil, Zestril), enalapril (Vasotec), and ramipril (Altace).

Angiotensin Receptor Blockers (ARBs): ARBs block the effects of angiotensin II, a hormone that constricts blood vessels and increases blood pressure. They have similar effects to ACE inhibitors and are often prescribed as an alternative for those who cannot tolerate ACE inhibitors. Commonly used ARBs include losartan (Cozaar), valsartan (Diovan), and candesartan (Atacand).

Beta-Blockers: Beta-blockers help slow the heart rate, reduce blood pressure, and improve heart function. They can decrease the workload on the heart and improve symptoms. Examples of beta-blockers commonly prescribed for CHF include carvedilol (Coreg), bisoprolol (Zebeta), and metoprolol (Lopressor, Toprol XL).

Aldosterone Antagonists: Aldosterone antagonists block the effects of the hormone aldosterone, which can contribute to fluid retention and worsen CHF symptoms. They can help reduce fluid buildup and improve heart function. Spironolactone (Aldactone) and eplerenone (Inspra) are common aldosterone antagonists used in CHF treatment.

Digoxin: Digoxin helps improve heart function and can be used to control heart rate in certain cases. It helps strengthen the heart's contractions and can alleviate symptoms such as fatigue and shortness of breath. Digoxin is often prescribed in combination with other medications.

Vasodilators: Vasodilators help relax and widen blood vessels, reducing the workload on the heart and improving blood flow. They can be used to alleviate symptoms and improve exercise tolerance. Examples include hydralazine (Apresoline) and isosorbide dinitrate (Isordil).

It's important to note that medication regimens for CHF may vary depending on individual factors, such as the severity of CHF, other underlying health conditions, and individual response to medications. Your healthcare provider will determine the most appropriate medications and dosages for your specific situation.

It's crucial to take medications as prescribed, follow up with your healthcare provider regularly, and report any side effects or concerns promptly. They will monitor your response to the medications and may make adjustments to the regimen as needed to optimize your treatment and improve your quality of life.

Understanding medication side effects

Understanding medication side effects is crucial for individuals taking medications for Congestive Heart Failure (CHF). While medications can effectively manage CHF symptoms and improve heart function, they can also potentially cause side effects. It's important to be aware of possible side effects and to promptly communicate any concerns to your healthcare provider. Here's some information to help you understand medication side effects:

Common Side Effects: Many medications used to treat CHF have common side effects that may occur in some individuals. These side effects can vary depending on the specific medication, dosage, and individual response. Some common side effects may include:

Diuretics: Increased urination, electrolyte imbalances (such as low potassium levels), dizziness, and dehydration.

ACE inhibitors and ARBs: Dry cough, low blood pressure, dizziness, increased potassium levels, and changes in kidney function.

Beta-blockers: Fatigue, dizziness, slowed heart rate, low blood pressure, and cold hands and feet.

Aldosterone antagonists: High potassium levels, changes in kidney function, and hormonal imbalances.

Digoxin: Nausea, vomiting, headache, dizziness, and visual disturbances.

Serious Side Effects: While less common, some medications may have serious side effects that require immediate medical attention. These can include:

Allergic reactions: Severe allergic reactions to medications can cause difficulty breathing, swelling of the face or throat, hives, or a rash. Seek immediate medical help if you experience these symptoms.

Irregular heart rhythms: Some medications can affect the electrical signals of the heart and may lead to irregular heart rhythms. Symptoms can include palpitations, dizziness, fainting, or chest pain. Contact your healthcare provider if you experience these symptoms.

Worsening kidney function: Certain medications can affect kidney function. If you notice changes in urination patterns, swelling in the legs or ankles, or persistent fatigue, inform your healthcare provider.

Liver problems: Rarely, some medications may cause liver problems. Watch for symptoms such as yellowing of the skin or eyes (jaundice), dark

urine, or persistent abdominal pain, and report them to your healthcare provider.
Communication with Healthcare Provider: It is essential to maintain open communication with your healthcare provider regarding any side effects you experience. They can assess the severity and determine the best course of action. Depending on the situation, they may adjust the medication dosage, switch to a different medication, or provide strategies to manage the side effects.

Adherence to Medication: Do not stop taking medications abruptly without consulting your healthcare provider, as this can have adverse effects. If you are experiencing side effects that are bothersome, discuss them with your healthcare provider, who can provide guidance on managing the side effects while ensuring effective CHF treatment.

Reporting Side Effects: If you experience any side effects, it is important to report them to your healthcare provider. They can document and monitor the side effects and adjust your treatment plan accordingly. Additionally, you can report side effects to the appropriate regulatory authorities, such as the Food and Drug Administration (FDA) in your country.

Remember, side effects can vary from person to person, and not everyone will experience them. By being vigilant, communicating openly with your healthcare provider, and following their guidance, you can effectively manage CHF treatment while minimizing the impact of medication side effects.

Importance of Regular Medical Check-up

Regular medical check-ups are of utmost importance for individuals living with Congestive Heart Failure (CHF). These check-ups provide an opportunity for healthcare providers to monitor your condition, assess treatment effectiveness, detect any potential complications or changes in your health, and make necessary adjustments to your care plan. Here are some key reasons why regular medical check-ups are essential:

Disease Progression Monitoring: CHF is a progressive condition, and regular check-ups allow your healthcare provider to monitor the progression of the disease. They can assess changes in your symptoms, evaluate your heart function through tests such as echocardiograms or electrocardiograms (ECGs), and determine if any modifications to your treatment plan are necessary.

Medication Management: Regular check-ups enable your healthcare provider to evaluate the effectiveness of your medication regimen. They can assess whether your medications are adequately controlling your symptoms, adjust dosages if needed, and monitor for any potential side effects or interactions with other medications.

Early Detection of Complications: CHF can lead to complications such as fluid retention, arrhythmias (abnormal heart rhythms), kidney dysfunction, or cardiac events. Regular check-ups allow healthcare providers to detect these complications early on through physical examinations, laboratory tests, and imaging studies. Early detection can lead to prompt intervention and treatment, potentially preventing further complications or hospitalizations.

Optimization of Treatment Plan: Each individual with CHF may have unique needs and responses to treatment. Regular check-ups provide an opportunity for your healthcare provider to assess your overall condition, review your lifestyle modifications, and ensure that your treatment plan is tailored to your specific needs. They can provide guidance on medication adherence, dietary changes, exercise routines, and stress management techniques to optimize your overall care.

Emotional and Psychological Support: Living with a chronic condition like CHF can be emotionally challenging. Regular check-ups allow for open discussions with your healthcare provider about your concerns, fears, and emotional well-being. They can provide support, address any mental health issues that may arise, and refer you to additional resources or specialists as needed.

Education and Empowerment: Regular check-ups are an opportunity to learn more about your condition and how to manage it effectively. Your healthcare provider can provide educational materials, explain test results, clarify any doubts or questions you may have, and empower you to take an active role in your self-care. By staying informed, you can make informed decisions about your lifestyle choices and treatment options.

Prevention and Health Promotion: Regular check-ups also focus on preventive measures and overall health promotion. Your healthcare provider may offer vaccinations, such as influenza or pneumococcal vaccines, to protect against respiratory infections that can exacerbate CHF symptoms. They may also provide guidance on maintaining a healthy weight, smoking cessation, alcohol moderation, and other lifestyle factors that can positively impact your heart health.

Remember, the frequency of check-ups may vary depending on your individual condition and healthcare provider's recommendations. Adhering to the scheduled check-ups and maintaining open communication with your healthcare provider are essential for effective CHF management and to ensure the best possible outcomes for your overall health and well-being.

Medical Procedures and Surgeries

In the management of Congestive Heart Failure (CHF), various medical procedures and surgeries may be recommended based on the individual's condition and specific needs. These procedures aim to improve heart function, alleviate symptoms, and prevent or treat complications. Here are some common medical procedures and surgeries used in the management of CHF:

Coronary Artery Bypass Grafting (CABG): CABG is a surgical procedure used to treat coronary artery disease, which often accompanies CHF. It involves bypassing blocked or narrowed coronary arteries by grafting healthy blood vessels from other parts of the body. By improving blood flow to the heart muscle, CABG can relieve chest pain (angina) and improve overall heart function.

Percutaneous Coronary Intervention (PCI): PCI, also known as angioplasty, is a minimally invasive procedure used to open blocked or narrowed coronary arteries. It involves inserting a catheter with a balloon at the tip into the affected artery and inflating the balloon to widen the artery. In some cases, a stent (a small mesh tube) is placed to help keep the artery open and improve blood flow.

Implantable Cardioverter-Defibrillator (ICD): An ICD is a device implanted in the chest to monitor and correct potentially life-threatening irregular heart rhythms. It continuously monitors the heart's electrical activity and can deliver electrical shocks or pacing to restore normal heart rhythm when needed. ICDs are often recommended for individuals at high risk of dangerous arrhythmias.

Cardiac Resynchronization Therapy (CRT): CRT, also known as biventricular pacing, is a procedure used for individuals with certain types of heart failure. It involves the implantation of a special pacemaker device that coordinates the contractions of the heart's chambers (ventricles) to improve overall pumping efficiency. CRT can help alleviate symptoms and improve heart function in selected individuals.

Ventricular Assist Devices (VADs): VADs are mechanical devices used to assist the pumping function of the heart in individuals with severe heart failure. These devices are implanted in the chest and can help maintain blood flow throughout the body while awaiting heart transplantation or as a long-term treatment option for those not eligible for transplantation.

Heart Transplantation: In severe cases of CHF, heart transplantation may be considered when other treatments have been ineffective. It involves replacing the diseased heart with a healthy heart from a deceased donor. Heart transplantation can significantly improve quality of life and long-term survival in carefully selected individuals. It's important to note that the decision to undergo a medical procedure or surgery depends on various factors, including the severity of CHF, overall health, and individual circumstances. The specific procedure or surgery recommended will be determined by a healthcare provider based on a thorough evaluation and discussion of the potential risks and benefits.

Each procedure has its own set of considerations, including potential complications, recovery time, and long-term implications. It is crucial to have detailed discussions with your healthcare provider, ask questions, and fully understand the procedure and its implications before making an informed decision.

Furthermore, it's important to have a multidisciplinary healthcare team, including cardiologists, cardiac surgeons, and specialized nurses, who will provide comprehensive care and support throughout the process of any medical procedure or surgery.

Navigating Everyday Life with CHF

Living with Congestive Heart Failure (CHF) requires adjustments to daily life to manage the condition effectively and maintain a good quality of life. Here are some strategies and tips to navigate everyday life with CHF:

Medication Adherence: Take your medications as prescribed by your healthcare provider. Set reminders, use pill organizers, and establish a routine to help ensure you take your medications consistently. If you have any concerns or difficulties with your medications, discuss them with your healthcare provider.

Lifestyle Modifications: Adopt heart-healthy lifestyle habits to support your overall well-being. This includes:

Following a balanced diet: Eat a diet rich in fruits, vegetables, whole grains, lean proteins, and low-fat dairy products. Limit sodium (salt) intake to help manage fluid retention.

Engaging in regular physical activity: Consult your healthcare provider for guidance on appropriate exercise routines. Physical activity can improve heart function, manage weight, and boost overall cardiovascular health.

Quitting smoking: Smoking can worsen CHF symptoms and increase the risk of complications. Seek support and resources to quit smoking if you're a smoker.

Limiting alcohol intake: Excessive alcohol consumption can strain the heart and interfere with medications. Discuss alcohol guidelines with your healthcare provider.

Fluid Management: Follow your healthcare provider's recommendations regarding fluid intake. Monitoring and managing fluid retention is crucial in CHF management. Be mindful of your fluid intake from beverages and foods, and consult your healthcare provider if you notice sudden weight gain or increased swelling.

Stress Management: Chronic stress can negatively impact heart health. Incorporate stress management techniques into your daily routine, such as deep breathing exercises, meditation, yoga, or engaging in hobbies and activities you enjoy. Seek support from friends, family, or professional counselors to help manage stress.

Regular Monitoring: Keep track of your symptoms, weight, blood pressure, and any changes in your condition. Regularly monitor your weight using a scale and report any significant changes to your healthcare provider, as it can indicate fluid retention.

Communication with Healthcare Provider: Maintain regular contact with your healthcare provider. Attend scheduled check-ups, discuss any concerns or changes in symptoms, and follow their recommendations for treatment adjustments or lifestyle modifications.

Support Network: Build a support network of family, friends, and support groups. Share your experiences, concerns, and successes with others who understand what you're going through. They can provide emotional support, encouragement, and practical assistance when needed.

Energy Conservation: Plan your activities wisely and prioritize tasks to conserve energy. Pace yourself throughout the day, take breaks when needed, and delegate tasks when possible. Listen to your body and rest when you feel fatigued.

Emergency Preparedness: Be prepared for emergencies by keeping a list of emergency contacts, understanding the signs of worsening symptoms, and having a plan in place for contacting medical professionals or seeking immediate medical attention when necessary.

Remember, each person's experience with CHF is unique, and it's important to work closely with your healthcare provider to tailor a management plan that suits your specific needs. By adopting a proactive approach to self-care, making necessary adjustments, and seeking support, you can effectively navigate everyday life with CHF and enhance your overall well-being.

Adapting to a New Normal

Adapting to a "new normal" after being diagnosed with Congestive Heart Failure (CHF) can be a challenging process, but it is possible to find a sense of stability and fulfillment in your life. Here are some strategies to help you adapt to your new normal:

Acceptance and Emotional Well-being: Accepting your diagnosis is an important step in adjusting to your new reality. Acknowledge your feelings and allow yourself to grieve the loss of your previous lifestyle. Seek support from loved ones, support groups, or professional counselors to help process your emotions and develop coping strategies.

Education and Knowledge: Learn as much as you can about CHF, its management, and available resources. Understanding your condition and treatment options empowers you to actively participate in your care and make informed decisions. Stay informed about the latest research, treatment advancements, and self-care techniques.

Self-Care and Prioritization: Prioritize self-care activities that promote your overall well-being. This includes following your treatment plan, engaging in regular physical activity (as recommended by your healthcare provider), getting adequate rest, eating a nutritious diet, and managing stress through relaxation techniques or hobbies you enjoy.

Establishing a Routine: Establish a daily routine that accommodates your CHF management needs. Incorporate medication schedules, dietary modifications, exercise routines, rest periods, and regular monitoring of symptoms into your routine. Having a structured schedule can provide a sense of control and stability.

Setting Realistic Goals: Set realistic goals that align with your current abilities and health condition. Break larger goals into smaller, achievable steps to maintain motivation and celebrate your progress. Focus on what you can do within your limitations rather than dwelling on what you cannot.

Open Communication: Communicate openly with your healthcare team, including doctors, nurses, and other healthcare professionals. Share any concerns, changes in symptoms, or challenges you are facing. They can provide guidance, make necessary adjustments to your treatment plan, and connect you with additional resources if needed.

Support Network: Surround yourself with a supportive network of family, friends, and peers who understand your journey. Seek support groups, both in-person and online, where you can connect with others living with CHF. Sharing experiences, advice, and encouragement can provide a sense of belonging and understanding.

Flexibility and Adaptability: Recognize that adapting to a new normal may require flexibility and adjustment along the way. Your health condition may fluctuate, and your needs may change over time. Be open to modifying your strategies, seeking new resources, and adjusting your expectations as necessary.

Celebrate Small Victories: Acknowledge and celebrate your achievements, no matter how small they may seem. Each step forward, each milestone reached, is an accomplishment. Recognize and appreciate your efforts and progress.

Adapting to a new normal takes time, patience, and resilience. Be kind to yourself, practice self-compassion, and celebrate the strengths and resilience you possess. With the right support, self-care practices, and a positive mindset, you can navigate your new normal with CHF and continue to live a fulfilling life.

Balancing Work and Lifestyle

Balancing work and lifestyle is crucial for individuals living with Congestive Heart Failure (CHF) to manage their condition effectively and maintain a good quality of life. Here are some strategies to help achieve a healthy balance:

Open Communication: Inform your employer or supervisor about your CHF diagnosis and any limitations or accommodations you may require. Discuss potential modifications to your work schedule or tasks that can support your health needs. Open communication fosters understanding and enables the creation of a work environment that promotes your well-being.

Prioritize Self-Care: Make self-care a priority. Take care of your physical and emotional well-being by following your treatment plan, getting enough rest, eating a nutritious diet, engaging in regular exercise (as recommended by your healthcare provider), and managing stress effectively. Remember that taking care of yourself is essential for managing your condition and maintaining your productivity at work.

Time Management: Practice effective time management to balance work tasks and personal activities. Prioritize your workload, set realistic deadlines, and break larger tasks into smaller, manageable steps. Use tools such as calendars, planners, or task management apps to stay organized and avoid overexertion.

Flexible Work Arrangements: Explore flexible work options that can accommodate your health needs. This may include working from home, adjusting work hours, or having the option to take breaks when needed. Discuss these possibilities with your employer or human resources department to find a solution that works for both parties.

Delegate and Seek Support: Delegate tasks when possible and ask for support from colleagues or supervisors. Recognize that you don't have to handle everything on your own. Delegating responsibilities can alleviate stress and ensure that work tasks are managed effectively while preserving your energy and well-being.

Work-Life Boundaries: Set clear boundaries between work and personal life. Avoid excessive overtime or bringing work-related stress into your personal time. Create dedicated spaces and times for relaxation, hobbies, spending time with loved ones, and engaging in activities that bring you joy and fulfillment.

Manage Stress: CHF management involves stress reduction. Implement stress management techniques, such as deep breathing exercises, meditation, or engaging in activities you enjoy outside of work. Practice stress-reducing techniques regularly to promote overall well-being.

Regular Breaks: Take regular breaks throughout the workday to rest and recharge. Short breaks can help alleviate physical and mental fatigue, improve focus, and enhance productivity. Use break times to engage in light stretching, walking, or other activities that promote circulation and relieve tension.

Healthy Work Environment: Create a supportive work environment by fostering positive relationships with colleagues and supervisors. Seek understanding and empathy from those around you. When possible, advocate for workplace policies and practices that support employee well-being and work-life balance.

Regular Check-Ups and Follow-Up: Keep up with your scheduled medical check-ups and follow-up appointments to ensure your condition is monitored and managed effectively. Proactively managing your health will minimize the risk of sudden exacerbation or hospitalization, allowing you to maintain stability in both work and personal life.

Finding the right balance between work and lifestyle is a personal journey. It may require trial and error, as well as ongoing adjustments. Listen to your body, communicate your needs, and be proactive in managing your condition. By prioritizing self-care and creating a supportive work environment, you can achieve a healthy balance that promotes both your professional success and overall well-being.

Traveling and Vacationing with CHF

Traveling and vacationing with Congestive Heart Failure (CHF) requires some extra planning and precautions to ensure a safe and enjoyable experience. Here are some tips to consider when traveling with CHF:

Consult Your Healthcare Provider: Before embarking on a trip, consult your healthcare provider to ensure you are medically stable for travel. Discuss your destination, mode of transportation, and the duration of your trip. Your healthcare provider can provide specific recommendations and precautions based on your individual health needs.

Plan Ahead: Research your destination and make necessary arrangements in advance. Consider factors such as climate, altitude, availability of medical facilities, and accessibility for individuals with mobility challenges. It's also important to check if your accommodations can accommodate any special needs or requirements.

Medications and Supplies: Ensure you have an ample supply of your medications for the duration of your trip, including any necessary prescriptions. Pack your medications in your carry-on bag to have them readily available during the journey. It may also be helpful to carry a written list of your medications, doses, and emergency contact information. Don't forget to bring any medical supplies or equipment you may need, such as a blood pressure monitor or a portable oxygen concentrator if required.

Stay Hydrated: Proper hydration is crucial when traveling with CHF. Carry a water bottle with you and drink plenty of fluids throughout your journey. Avoid excessive intake of caffeinated or alcoholic beverages, as they can contribute to dehydration. If you have fluid restrictions, consult your healthcare provider for specific guidelines regarding fluid intake while traveling.

Pace Yourself: Take your time and pace yourself during your trip. Allow for plenty of rest periods and avoid overexertion. Plan activities and sightseeing in a way that allows for breaks and periods of relaxation. Be mindful of your energy levels and listen to your body.

Watch Your Diet: Pay attention to your diet while traveling, especially when it comes to sodium (salt) intake. Limit your consumption of high-sodium foods, as excessive sodium can contribute to fluid retention and worsen CHF symptoms. Opt for healthier food choices, such as fresh fruits, vegetables, and lean proteins. If dining out, ask for low-sodium options or request that your meals be prepared without added salt.

Maintain a Healthy Lifestyle: Stick to your regular CHF management routine as much as possible while traveling. This includes following your prescribed exercise regimen, monitoring your weight, and adhering to dietary guidelines. Stay consistent with your medication schedule and don't skip doses.

Stay Prepared for Emergencies: Carry a list of emergency contact numbers, including your healthcare provider's information and any local medical facilities at your destination. Familiarize yourself with the nearest medical facilities and emergency services. Consider purchasing travel insurance that covers medical emergencies to provide peace of mind during your trip.

Travel Companions: Consider traveling with a companion, especially if you have specific care needs or require assistance. Having someone by your side can provide support, help with logistics, and offer assistance in case of an emergency.

Take Breaks from Travel: If you're embarking on a long journey, consider breaking it up with layovers or stopping points to allow for rest and recovery. Prolonged sitting or immobility during travel can increase the risk of blood clots. When flying, try to move and stretch your legs periodically to promote circulation.

Remember to listen to your body and prioritize your well-being throughout your trip. Be mindful of your limitations and adjust your activities accordingly. With proper planning, precautions, and adherence to your CHF management plan, you can enjoy safe and memorable travel experiences.

Tips for Managing Medications and Doctor Appointments

Managing medications and doctor appointments is crucial for individuals with Congestive Heart Failure (CHF) to effectively manage their condition. Here are some tips to help you stay organized and ensure you are on track with your medications and appointments:

Create a Medication Schedule: Develop a medication schedule that outlines the names of your medications, dosages, and specific times for taking each medication. This can be in the form of a written chart, a digital reminder on your phone, or a medication management app. Having a clear schedule will help you remember when to take your medications and avoid missed doses.

Use Medication Reminders: Set up reminders to alert you when it's time to take your medications. This can be done using alarm clocks, smartphone apps, or medication reminder devices. Choose a method that works best for you and ensures you stay on track with your medication regimen.

Organize Medications: Keep your medications organized in pill organizers or medication containers labeled with the days of the week and specific times. This will help you easily identify which medications to take and when. Consider using separate organizers for morning, afternoon, and evening doses to avoid confusion.

Take Medications as Prescribed: Follow your healthcare provider's instructions regarding medication dosage and frequency. Avoid skipping doses or adjusting medication doses without consulting your healthcare provider first. If you have any concerns or questions about your medications, discuss them with your healthcare provider or pharmacist.

Keep a Medication List: Maintain an updated list of all your medications, including prescription drugs, over-the-counter medications, and supplements. Include the names, dosages, and instructions for each medication. Keep a copy of this list in your wallet or purse, and provide a copy to your healthcare provider during appointments or hospital visits.

Refill Medications on Time: Stay proactive about refilling your medications to ensure you don't run out. Set reminders to refill prescriptions a few days before they are due to run out. Consider using mail-order pharmacy services or automatic prescription refills to streamline the process.

Stay Organized with Doctor Appointments: Keep track of your upcoming doctor appointments by maintaining a calendar specifically for healthcare-related appointments. Note the date, time, and location of each appointment. Set reminders a few days before each appointment to ensure you are prepared and don't miss them.

Prepare for Doctor Appointments: Before each appointment, prepare a list of questions or concerns you want to discuss with your healthcare provider. Include any changes in symptoms, side effects of medications, or other issues you may have encountered. Bring along your medication list and any relevant medical records or test results.

Communicate with Your Healthcare Team: Maintain open communication with your healthcare team. Inform them about any changes in your symptoms, medication side effects, or other health concerns. Regularly follow up with your healthcare provider to address any questions or issues that arise.

Utilize Technology: Take advantage of technology to streamline medication management and appointment scheduling. Use smartphone apps or online platforms that allow you to track medications, set reminders, and schedule doctor appointments. Some platforms even offer the ability to communicate with your healthcare provider electronically.

Remember, proper medication management and regular doctor appointments are essential for effectively managing your CHF. By staying organized, utilizing reminders, and maintaining open communication with your healthcare team, you can ensure that you are on track with your medications and receive the necessary care to keep your condition well-managed.

Relationships and Emotional Well-being

Relationships and emotional well-being play a vital role in managing Congestive Heart Failure (CHF) and maintaining a positive outlook on life. Here are some tips for nurturing relationships and supporting your emotional well-being:

Communicate Openly: Maintain open and honest communication with your loved ones about your CHF diagnosis, treatment, and any challenges you may face. Express your feelings, fears, and concerns. Effective communication helps your loved ones understand your needs and allows them to offer support.

Seek Support: Reach out to friends, family, and support groups who can provide emotional support and understanding. Share your experiences with others who may have gone through similar situations. Online communities and local support groups can provide a safe space for sharing and receiving support.

Educate Loved Ones: Help your family and friends understand CHF by providing them with educational resources. This can help them comprehend your condition better and foster empathy and support.

Emotional Coping Strategies: Develop healthy coping strategies to manage stress, anxiety, and any emotional challenges that may arise due to your CHF diagnosis. These can include relaxation techniques, mindfulness exercises, deep breathing exercises, journaling, or engaging in activities that bring you joy and peace.

Professional Counseling: Consider seeking professional counseling or therapy to address emotional well-being. A therapist can provide guidance, tools, and support in managing emotions related to CHF, helping you navigate the challenges that may arise.

Maintain Social Connections: Stay connected with friends and loved ones, even if physical limitations or fatigue make it challenging. Regular social interactions can help combat feelings of isolation and boost emotional well-being. Consider engaging in activities that you enjoy, such as going for walks, having meals together, or participating in hobbies with loved ones.

Practice Self-Care: Prioritize self-care to support your emotional well-being. Engage in activities that promote relaxation, reduce stress, and bring you joy. This can include hobbies, reading, listening to music, spending time in nature, or practicing meditation or yoga. Taking care of your physical health, such as getting adequate rest and eating a balanced diet, also contributes to your emotional well-being.

Emotional Boundaries: Set emotional boundaries with loved ones and caregivers to ensure your emotional well-being is protected. Communicate your needs and limitations, and be assertive in expressing what you are comfortable with in terms of emotional support.

Celebrate Milestones and Victories: Recognize and celebrate your personal milestones and victories, no matter how small they may seem. This can help boost your self-esteem, enhance your sense of accomplishment, and foster a positive outlook.

Accept and Express Emotions: Allow yourself to experience a range of emotions that may arise due to your CHF diagnosis. Give yourself permission to grieve, be angry, or feel frustrated at times. Expressing your emotions in a healthy way, such as through journaling or talking to a trusted friend or therapist, can be therapeutic and help you navigate your emotional journey.

Remember, maintaining strong relationships and supporting your emotional well-being are essential components of managing CHF. By nurturing your relationships, seeking support, practicing self-care, and addressing your emotional needs, you can enhance your overall well-being and resilience in the face of CHF.

Communicating with Loved Ones about CHF

Communicating with loved ones about your Congestive Heart Failure (CHF) diagnosis is essential for building understanding, fostering support, and strengthening your relationships. Here are some tips to help you effectively communicate with your loved ones about CHF:

Choose the Right Time and Place: Find a comfortable and appropriate setting to have open and honest conversations about your CHF. Ensure there are minimal distractions and enough time for a meaningful discussion.

Be Prepared: Before initiating a conversation, gather relevant information about CHF, including its symptoms, treatments, and lifestyle changes. This will help you provide accurate and detailed information to your loved ones, answering any questions they may have.

Explain CHF Clearly: Start by explaining what CHF is in simple terms. Describe how it affects the heart's functioning, the symptoms you experience, and how it impacts your daily life. Provide examples that help your loved ones understand the challenges you face.

Share Your Feelings and Experiences: Express your emotions, fears, and concerns about living with CHF. Help your loved ones understand the impact it has on your physical and emotional well-being. Sharing your experiences will give them insight into your journey and foster empathy.

Encourage Questions and Listen: Encourage your loved ones to ask questions and express their concerns. Be patient and attentive as they share their thoughts and emotions. Listening actively shows that you value their perspective and encourages open dialogue.

Provide Educational Resources: Share educational materials, such as brochures, websites, or books, that explain CHF in more detail. These resources can help your loved ones gain a better understanding of the condition and its implications.

Discuss Lifestyle Changes: Talk about the lifestyle changes recommended for managing CHF, such as dietary modifications, exercise routines, and medication adherence. Explain how these changes contribute to your overall well-being and may impact your daily activities.

Clarify Support Needs: Communicate your specific support needs to your loved ones. Be clear about how they can assist you, whether it's accompanying you to medical appointments, helping with household chores, or offering emotional support. Encourage open dialogue to determine what types of support are most helpful to you.

Address Misconceptions: Correct any misconceptions or myths that your loved ones may have about CHF. Provide accurate information to dispel misunderstandings and ensure everyone is on the same page.

Express Appreciation: Show gratitude for the support and understanding your loved ones offer. Let them know that their presence and involvement in your CHF journey mean a lot to you. Acknowledge their efforts and express how their support positively impacts your well-being.

Remember that open and ongoing communication is key to maintaining strong relationships. Continue to have regular conversations with your loved ones about your experiences, updates on your health, and any changes in your condition. By fostering a supportive and understanding environment, you can strengthen your relationships and navigate CHF together.

Intimacy and Sexual Health

Intimacy and sexual health are important aspects of overall well-being, and living with Congestive Heart Failure (CHF) may introduce unique considerations in this area. Here are some tips for addressing intimacy and sexual health while managing CHF:

Open Communication: Communicate openly and honestly with your partner about your feelings, concerns, and any physical limitations or symptoms you experience due to CHF. Share your needs, desires, and fears related to intimacy and sexual activity. This open dialogue can help build understanding and strengthen your emotional connection.

Involve Your Healthcare Team: Discuss any concerns or questions about intimacy and sexual health with your healthcare provider. They can provide guidance tailored to your specific health condition and offer recommendations for managing CHF-related symptoms during sexual activity.

Educate Yourself: Learn about the potential impact of CHF on sexual health and intimacy. Understand the physical limitations or precautions you may need to consider. Knowledge empowers you to make informed decisions and communicate effectively with your partner.

Pace Yourself: Take things at a pace that is comfortable for you. Listen to your body and be mindful of any symptoms or signs of fatigue during intimate moments. Rest and take breaks as needed. Finding a balance between physical activity and rest can help manage symptoms and maintain intimacy.

Explore Different Intimate Activities: Sexual intimacy involves more than just sexual intercourse. Explore alternative forms of intimacy that focus on emotional connection, such as cuddling, holding hands, kissing, or gentle touching. Engaging in these activities can strengthen the bond with your partner.

Modify Positions: If certain sexual positions are uncomfortable or physically challenging, consider trying different positions that are more comfortable and put less strain on your heart and body. Experiment with positions that allow you to maintain comfort and minimize physical exertion.

Consider Timing: Plan sexual activity at times when you feel most rested and have the least amount of symptoms. This may vary for each individual, so listen to your body and choose the right time for you.

Manage Medications: Some medications used to manage CHF may affect sexual function. If you experience any side effects that impact your sexual health, discuss them with your healthcare provider. They may adjust your medication regimen or suggest alternative options to minimize the impact on your sexual well-being.

Emotional Support: Seek emotional support from your partner, as well as from support groups or counseling services specializing in sexual health and intimacy. Connecting with others who have similar experiences can provide a safe space for sharing and receiving support.

Consult a Specialist: If you have persistent concerns or difficulties related to sexual health or intimacy, consider consulting a healthcare professional who specializes in sexual medicine or a therapist experienced in addressing these issues. They can provide personalized guidance and support tailored to your needs.

Remember, intimacy and sexual health are unique to each individual, and it's important to prioritize your comfort, well-being, and emotional connection with your partner. By maintaining open communication, seeking appropriate support, and adapting to your physical limitations, you can nurture intimacy and maintain a fulfilling and satisfying relationship while managing CHF.

Coping with Emotional Challenges

Coping with emotional challenges is an important aspect of living with Congestive Heart Failure (CHF) as it can significantly impact your overall well-being. Here are some strategies to help you effectively cope with emotional challenges:

Acknowledge and Accept Your Feelings: Allow yourself to acknowledge and accept the range of emotions you may experience, such as fear, sadness, frustration, or anxiety. Recognize that it is normal to have these feelings and that they are valid. Give yourself permission to feel and process them.

Seek Support: Reach out to your support network, including friends, family, or support groups, to share your emotions and concerns. Talking to others who understand or have experienced similar challenges can provide validation, empathy, and practical advice.

Engage in Self-Care: Prioritize self-care activities that promote emotional well-being. This can include engaging in hobbies, practicing relaxation techniques like deep breathing or meditation, exercising regularly, getting enough restful sleep, and maintaining a balanced diet. Taking care of yourself physically can positively impact your emotional state.

Practice Stress Management Techniques: Develop and incorporate stress management techniques into your daily routine. This can include activities like yoga, mindfulness, guided imagery, or journaling. Engaging in these practices can help reduce stress levels and promote emotional balance.

Maintain a Positive Mindset: Cultivate a positive mindset by focusing on gratitude and positive aspects of your life. Practice reframing negative thoughts into more positive and empowering ones. Surround yourself with uplifting and supportive people and engage in activities that bring joy and happiness.

Educate Yourself: Gain knowledge about CHF and its management. Understanding your condition and treatment options can help alleviate fears and empower you to take an active role in your health. Talk to your healthcare provider, attend educational programs, or read reputable resources to enhance your understanding.

Set Realistic Goals: Set achievable goals that are aligned with your capabilities and current circumstances. Breaking down larger goals into smaller, manageable steps can make them more attainable and provide a sense of accomplishment.

Seek Professional Help: If emotional challenges become overwhelming or persist over an extended period, consider seeking professional help. A therapist or counselor can provide guidance, support, and strategies to help you cope with specific emotional challenges related to CHF.

Practice Mindfulness and Emotional Awareness: Stay present in the moment and practice mindfulness. Pay attention to your emotions and thoughts without judgment. This awareness can help you identify triggers and develop healthier responses to emotional challenges.

Give Yourself Grace: Be compassionate with yourself and practice self-compassion. Recognize that living with CHF can be challenging, and it's okay to have difficult days. Treat yourself with kindness and patience, celebrating your resilience and progress along the way.

Remember that coping with emotional challenges is an ongoing process, and it's important to be gentle with yourself as you navigate the ups and downs of living with CHF. Implementing these strategies and seeking appropriate support can help you build emotional resilience and improve your overall well-being.

Seeking Professional Mental Health Support

Seeking professional mental health support is an important step in managing the emotional challenges that can accompany living with Congestive Heart Failure (CHF). Here are some considerations and steps to help you in seeking professional help:

Recognize the Need: If you are experiencing persistent feelings of sadness, anxiety, depression, or if emotional challenges are significantly impacting your daily functioning and quality of life, it may be a sign that professional mental health support is needed.

Consult with Your Healthcare Provider: Start by discussing your concerns with your primary healthcare provider or cardiologist. They can evaluate your overall health, assess your emotional well-being, and provide recommendations or referrals to mental health professionals who specialize in working with individuals managing chronic health conditions like CHF.

Research and Find a Suitable Mental Health Professional: Look for mental health professionals who have experience or expertise in working with individuals coping with chronic illnesses or medical conditions. This can include psychologists, psychiatrists, licensed therapists, or counselors. Consider factors such as their credentials, experience, approach, and compatibility with your needs.

Reach Out for Appointments: Contact mental health professionals you have identified to inquire about their availability and schedule an appointment. Some mental health professionals may have specific expertise in health psychology or counseling for individuals with chronic illnesses, which can be beneficial in addressing the unique challenges of living with CHF.

Prepare for Your Appointment: Before your appointment, prepare a list of questions or concerns you would like to discuss. Reflect on your emotional experiences, symptoms, and any specific challenges you have faced. This will help guide the conversation and ensure that you cover all relevant aspects during your session.

Be Open and Honest: During your appointment, be open and honest about your experiences, emotions, and challenges. Share any specific concerns you have related to living with CHF and how it affects your emotional well-being. This information will assist the mental health professional in developing an appropriate treatment plan tailored to your needs.

Follow the Treatment Plan: Work collaboratively with your mental health professional to develop a treatment plan that addresses your specific emotional challenges. This may involve individual therapy, cognitive-behavioral therapy (CBT), medication management, or other evidence-based interventions. Follow through with the recommendations and actively participate in the therapeutic process.

Maintain Communication: Stay in regular contact with your mental health professional, keeping them informed of any changes or updates regarding your emotional well-being. If you have any concerns or questions between appointments, don't hesitate to reach out for clarification or support.

Explore Support Groups: In addition to individual therapy, consider joining support groups or counseling programs specifically designed for individuals managing chronic illnesses or heart conditions. These groups can provide additional support, understanding, and a sense of community.

Remember that seeking professional mental health support is a sign of strength and a proactive step towards managing your emotional well-being. Mental health professionals can provide you with valuable tools, strategies, and support to navigate the emotional challenges associated with living with CHF.

Overcoming Obstacles and Achieving Dreams

Overcoming obstacles and achieving your dreams while living with Congestive Heart Failure (CHF) requires determination, resilience, and a positive mindset. Here are some strategies to help you navigate challenges and work towards your goals:

Set Realistic Goals: Identify your dreams and break them down into smaller, manageable goals. Setting realistic and achievable goals allows you to make progress step by step and maintain motivation along the way.

Embrace a Growth Mindset: Adopt a mindset that views challenges as opportunities for growth and learning. See setbacks as temporary and use them as fuel to come back stronger. Believe in your ability to overcome obstacles and persevere despite the challenges.

Seek Support: Surround yourself with a supportive network of friends, family, or fellow CHF patients who understand and encourage your aspirations. Seek their guidance, advice, and emotional support when facing obstacles. Their encouragement can help fuel your determination.

Take Care of Your Physical and Emotional Well-being: Prioritize self-care to maintain your physical and emotional health. Follow your treatment plan, engage in regular exercise, eat a balanced diet, get enough restful sleep, and manage stress effectively. Taking care of your well-being provides you with the energy and resilience needed to overcome obstacles.

Adapt and Adjust: Be open to adapting your goals and plans as needed. CHF may require you to make adjustments along the way, but it doesn't mean you have to give up on your dreams. Be flexible, explore alternative paths, and find creative solutions that align with your current abilities and circumstances.

Break Down Barriers: Identify the specific obstacles that stand in your way and brainstorm strategies to overcome them. Whether it's physical limitations, financial constraints, or time constraints, seek solutions and resources that can help you overcome these barriers. Research available support programs, financial assistance, or adaptive technologies that can aid in pursuing your dreams.

Educate Yourself and Seek Opportunities: Stay informed about resources, opportunities, and advancements related to CHF and your field of interest. Attend workshops, seminars, or webinars to enhance your knowledge and skills. Seek out opportunities to engage in activities aligned with your dreams, such as volunteering, internships, or part-time work in your desired field.

Cultivate Resilience: Develop resilience by viewing challenges as opportunities for growth and learning. Reframe setbacks as valuable lessons that can propel you forward. Develop coping strategies to bounce back from setbacks and setbacks and develop a resilient mindset that helps you persevere.

Celebrate Milestones and Small Victories: Acknowledge and celebrate your progress along the way. Each milestone and small victory brings you closer to your dreams. Recognize and appreciate the effort, determination, and resilience you demonstrate, regardless of the size of the achievement.

Stay Focused on Your Passion: Stay connected to your passion and purpose. Remind yourself why your dreams matter to you and how they contribute to your overall well-being and happiness. Let your passion fuel your motivation and keep you moving forward, even in the face of obstacles.

Remember, your dreams are within reach, and CHF does not define your potential. With perseverance, adaptability, and a positive mindset, you can overcome obstacles, navigate challenges, and achieve your dreams. Stay committed to your goals, seek support, and believe in your ability to create a fulfilling and meaningful life, despite the challenges you may face.

Celebrating Life's Victories, Big and Small

Celebrating life's victories, big and small, is an essential practice that can bring joy, gratitude, and motivation into your life, especially while managing Congestive Heart Failure (CHF). Here are some ways to celebrate and acknowledge your victories:

Recognize the Importance of Small Wins: Don't underestimate the power of small victories. Celebrate even the smallest milestones and achievements along your journey. Whether it's completing a task, sticking to your treatment plan, or accomplishing a personal goal, take a moment to acknowledge and appreciate these accomplishments.

Practice Gratitude: Cultivate a sense of gratitude for the blessings in your life. Take time each day to reflect on the positive aspects, no matter how small they may seem. Express gratitude for your health, the support of loved ones, the beauty of nature, or any other elements that bring you joy and positivity.

Create a Celebration Ritual: Establish a personal celebration ritual to mark significant achievements. It could be as simple as treating yourself to a special meal, enjoying a relaxing spa day, or engaging in an activity you love. The important thing is to create a meaningful and enjoyable way to acknowledge your victories.

Share Your Triumphs: Share your accomplishments with loved ones, friends, or support groups. Celebrating with others who understand and support you can enhance the joy and create a sense of community. Their encouragement and applause can boost your confidence and motivation.

Record Your Successes: Keep a journal or create a "victory board" to record your achievements, both big and small. Write down the milestones you have reached, the obstacles you have overcome, and the positive experiences you have had. When you need a reminder of how far you've come, revisit these records to feel a sense of pride and accomplishment.

Reflect on Lessons Learned: Celebrate not only the outcome but also the process. Take time to reflect on the lessons and growth you have experienced throughout your journey. Recognize the skills you have developed, the resilience you have shown, and the personal insights gained. Embrace the learning opportunities that come with each victory.

Treat Yourself with Self-Compassion: Be kind to yourself and practice self-compassion. Celebrating your victories involves acknowledging your efforts and progress, even if the results may not always be perfect. Treat yourself with patience, understanding, and forgiveness. Remember that setbacks are a part of life, and every step forward is worth celebrating.

Embrace the Power of Positive Affirmations: Use positive affirmations to reinforce your belief in yourself and your ability to overcome challenges. Repeat affirmations that align with your achievements and goals. For example, affirm statements like, "I am strong, resilient, and capable of achieving my dreams.

Share Inspiring Stories: Engage with others who have faced similar challenges and share inspiring stories of triumph and resilience. Celebrate their victories and draw inspiration from their experiences. By celebrating the achievements of others, you cultivate a culture of positivity and support.

Live in the Present Moment: Practice mindfulness and savor each moment. Celebrate the present moment by fully immersing yourself in the experience. Appreciate the progress you have made and find joy in the present rather than constantly focusing on future goals.

Remember, celebrating life's victories, big and small, is not only about the outcome but also about acknowledging your efforts, growth, and resilience. Embrace the journey and celebrate yourself along the way, as each victory brings you closer to living a fulfilling and meaningful life with CHF.

Looking Forward to the Future

Looking forward to the future is an important mindset to cultivate while living with Congestive Heart Failure (CHF). Despite the challenges you may face, maintaining a positive outlook and embracing the possibilities that lie ahead can bring hope, motivation, and a sense of purpose. Here are some strategies to help you look forward to the future:

Set Goals and Dreams: Identify your goals, aspirations, and dreams for the future. Whether they are related to your personal life, relationships, career, or hobbies, having something to look forward to can provide a sense of direction and purpose. Set realistic and meaningful goals that align with your abilities and values.

Create a Vision Board: Visualize your ideal future by creating a vision board. Gather images, quotes, and symbols that represent the life you envision for yourself. Display this vision board in a prominent place where you can see it daily. It will serve as a reminder of your dreams and inspire you to take steps towards realizing them.

Practice Positive Visualization: Dedicate time each day to visualize yourself living the life you desire. Imagine yourself achieving your goals, experiencing joy, and embracing a fulfilling future. Engage all your senses in this visualization process to make it vivid and emotionally impactful. This practice can fuel your motivation and reinforce a positive mindset.

Cultivate Optimism: Develop an optimistic outlook on life. Focus on the possibilities and opportunities that lie ahead rather than dwelling on limitations or setbacks. Surround yourself with positive influences, such as uplifting books, inspiring stories, or motivational speakers, to help maintain an optimistic mindset.

Embrace Self-Care: Take care of your physical, emotional, and mental well-being. Engage in activities that bring you joy, relaxation, and rejuvenation. Prioritize self-care practices that nourish and energize you, whether it's spending time in nature, practicing mindfulness, engaging in creative pursuits, or enjoying quality time with loved ones.

Stay Engaged and Connected: Seek opportunities for engagement and connection with others. Participate in support groups, community activities, or social gatherings that align with your interests and values. Building meaningful relationships and maintaining a sense of community can provide support, inspiration, and a shared sense of purpose.

Continuously Learn and Grow: Cultivate a mindset of continuous learning and personal growth. Engage in activities that expand your knowledge, develop new skills, or explore new hobbies. Consider taking online courses, attending workshops, or joining clubs or organizations that align with your interests. Embracing lifelong learning keeps your mind active and opens doors to new possibilities.

Stay Informed about CHF Advancement: Keep yourself informed about the latest advancements, research, and treatment options related to CHF. Stay in touch with your healthcare provider and discuss any new developments that may be relevant to your condition. Knowing that advancements are being made in the field can provide hope for improved treatment options and quality of life.

Nurture Supportive Relationships: Surround yourself with supportive and understanding individuals who uplift and encourage you. Build a network of friends, family, or fellow CHF patients who can provide emotional support, share experiences, and inspire each other. Having a strong support system can help you face challenges and look forward to the future with confidence.

Practice Mindfulness and Gratitude: Stay present in the moment and cultivate a sense of gratitude for the blessings in your life. Appreciate the small joys, positive experiences, and progress you make along your journey. Mindfulness and gratitude practices can help you stay grounded, reduce anxiety, and foster a positive outlook.

Remember that looking forward to the future is about embracing hope, resilience, and a belief in your ability to create a meaningful and fulfilling life. Despite the challenges of CHF, there are still countless possibilities and opportunities waiting for you. Stay focused on your dreams, take proactive steps towards your goals, and have faith in your ability to shape a future that brings you happiness, fulfillment, and a sense of purpose.

Promising Research and Achievements in CHF

There have been promising research developments and achievements in the field of Congestive Heart Failure (CHF) that offer hope for improved treatments and outcomes. Here are some notable advancements:

Precision Medicine: Researchers are increasingly focusing on precision medicine, which involves tailoring treatment strategies based on an individual's unique genetic and molecular characteristics. This approach aims to optimize treatment effectiveness and reduce adverse effects by providing targeted therapies specific to each patient's needs.

Advances in Drug Therapies: Several new medications have been developed and approved for the treatment of CHF. These include angiotensin receptor-neprilysin inhibitors (ARNIs), which have shown significant benefits in reducing hospitalizations and mortality rates in patients with reduced ejection fraction. Other medications, such as SGLT2 inhibitors and guanylate cyclase stimulators, have also demonstrated positive outcomes in clinical trials.

Cardiac Resynchronization Therapy (CRT): CRT, also known as biventricular pacing, has been shown to improve the quality of life and survival rates in patients with advanced heart failure and electrical dyssynchrony. This therapy involves the implantation of a device that coordinates the contraction of the heart's chambers, optimizing its pumping efficiency.

Mechanical Circulatory Support: Technological advancements in mechanical circulatory support devices, such as left ventricular assist devices (LVADs) and total artificial hearts, have improved the survival and quality of life for patients with end-stage heart failure. These devices can help bridge patients to heart transplantation or serve as a long-term therapy option.

Stem Cell Therapy: Researchers are exploring the potential of stem cell therapy to regenerate damaged heart tissue and improve heart function in CHF patients. Early studies have shown promising results, indicating the potential for future breakthroughs in this field.

Telemedicine and Remote Monitoring: The integration of telemedicine and remote monitoring technologies has enhanced the management of CHF by allowing healthcare providers to monitor patients' vital signs, symptoms, and medication adherence remotely. This approach can help identify early warning signs, prevent complications, and provide timely interventions, leading to improved outcomes.

Artificial Intelligence (AI) and Machine Learning: AI and machine learning algorithms are being developed to analyze vast amounts of patient data and predict CHF exacerbations, hospital readmissions, and treatment responses. These predictive models can help guide personalized treatment plans and improve patient outcomes.

Patient Education and Self-Management Programs: There is growing recognition of the importance of patient education and self-management programs in CHF management. These programs empower patients with knowledge about their condition, lifestyle modifications, medication adherence, and symptom recognition. By actively participating in their care, patients can better manage their condition and improve their quality of life.

Collaborative Research Efforts: Various organizations, research institutions, and pharmaceutical companies are collaborating on large-scale clinical trials and research initiatives to advance our understanding of CHF and develop innovative treatment approaches. These collaborative efforts bring together expertise from different fields, accelerating progress in CHF research.

It's important to note that while these advancements are promising, further research and clinical trials are needed to validate their long-term efficacy and safety. Nevertheless, these achievements offer hope for better outcomes and

improved quality of life for individuals
living with CHF.

Maintaining Long-term Health and Wellness

Maintaining long-term health and wellness is crucial for individuals living with Congestive Heart Failure (CHF). While CHF presents challenges, there are several key strategies that can help promote overall well-being and support a healthier lifestyle. Here are some important considerations:

Follow a Heart-Healthy Diet: Adopting a heart-healthy diet can significantly contribute to your long-term health. Focus on consuming nutrient-rich foods such as fruits, vegetables, whole grains, lean proteins, and healthy fats. Limit your intake of sodium, saturated fats, and processed foods. Consult with a registered dietitian or healthcare provider to develop a personalized meal plan that suits your specific dietary needs and restrictions.

Engage in Regular Physical Activity: Regular exercise plays a vital role in maintaining cardiovascular health. Consult with your healthcare provider to determine a suitable exercise regimen based on your individual capabilities and limitations. Engage in aerobic exercises, such as walking, swimming, or cycling, which can improve cardiovascular fitness. Incorporate strength training exercises to maintain muscle mass and enhance overall physical function.

Manage Fluid Intake: Fluid management is crucial for individuals with CHF, as excessive fluid retention can strain the heart. Follow your healthcare provider's recommendations for monitoring and regulating fluid intake. Limit your sodium intake, as it can contribute to fluid retention. Keep track of your daily fluid intake and weigh yourself regularly to detect any sudden changes that may require medical attention.

Adhere to Medication and Treatment Plans: Strict adherence to prescribed medications, including heart medications, diuretics, and other treatments, is essential for managing CHF effectively. Follow your healthcare provider's instructions regarding dosage, timing, and potential side effects. If you experience any concerns or difficulties with your medications, consult your healthcare provider promptly.

Monitor and Manage Symptoms: Stay vigilant about monitoring your symptoms and promptly report any changes or concerns to your healthcare provider. Regularly measure your blood pressure, monitor your weight, and track any symptoms such as shortness of breath, fatigue, or swelling. Adhere to your healthcare provider's recommendations for self-care measures and seek medical attention when necessary.

Reduce Stress: Chronic stress can negatively impact heart health. Practice stress management techniques such as deep breathing exercises, meditation, yoga, or engaging in activities that bring you joy and relaxation. Seek support from loved ones, join support groups, or consider therapy or counseling to help manage stress effectively.

Get Sufficient Rest and Sleep: Prioritize getting enough rest and quality sleep to support overall well-being. Aim for 7-8 hours of sleep each night and establish a regular sleep routine. If you experience sleep disturbances, such as sleep apnea or insomnia, consult with your healthcare provider for appropriate management strategies.

Quit Smoking and Limit Alcohol Intake: If you smoke, quitting is essential for your cardiovascular health. Smoking cessation can significantly reduce the risk of further damage to your heart and blood vessels. Additionally, limit alcohol intake, as excessive alcohol consumption can negatively impact heart health and interact with medications.

Regular Medical Check-ups: Maintain regular follow-up appointments with your healthcare provider to monitor your condition, assess treatment effectiveness, and make necessary adjustments to your care plan. Routine check-ups, including physical examinations, laboratory tests, and diagnostic imaging, can help detect any changes or complications early on.
Emotional and Mental Well-being: Pay attention to your emotional and mental well-being. Seek support from loved ones, join support groups, or consider therapy or counseling if you are experiencing emotional challenges or mental health concerns. Engage in

activities that bring you joy, practice self-care, and prioritize self-compassion.

Remember, maintaining long-term health and wellness with CHF requires a holistic approach that encompasses physical, emotional, and mental well-being. By incorporating these strategies into your lifestyle and working closely with your healthcare team, you can optimize your health, improve quality of life, and manage CHF more effectively.

Advocacy and Support for CHF Awareness

Advocacy and support for Congestive Heart Failure (CHF) awareness are crucial in raising public consciousness about the condition, promoting early detection and intervention, and improving the quality of life for individuals living with CHF. Here are some ways you can get involved in advocacy and support efforts:

1. **Join Support Groups**: Connect with local or online support groups specifically focused on CHF. These groups provide a platform for sharing experiences, exchanging information, and offering support to one another. Participating in support groups can help you navigate the challenges of CHF while also gaining insights and emotional support from individuals who understand your journey.

2. **Volunteer for CHF Organizations**: Many organizations dedicated to heart health and CHF provide volunteer opportunities. You can contribute your time and skills to support their initiatives, such as fundraising events, awareness campaigns, community education programs, or patient support activities. Volunteering allows you to make a meaningful impact in the CHF community and raise awareness about the condition.

3. **Advocate for Policy Change**: Get involved in advocacy efforts aimed at influencing policy changes related to CHF. This may involve contacting local representatives, participating in awareness campaigns, or joining advocacy organizations that focus on cardiovascular health. By advocating for improved access to healthcare, research funding, and support services, you can

help create a more favorable environment for individuals living with CHF.

4. **Share Your Story**: Personal stories have a powerful impact in raising awareness and inspiring others. Consider sharing your experience with CHF through various channels, such as social media, blogs, or local publications. By sharing your journey, challenges, and triumphs, you can provide hope and encouragement to others facing similar situations and help reduce the stigma associated with CHF.

5. **Participate in Research Studies**: Contributing to research studies and clinical trials can advance our understanding of CHF and lead to improved treatment options. Explore opportunities to participate in research studies related to CHF at local universities, research institutions, or hospitals. Your participation can help

researchers gather valuable data and insights that can shape the future of CHF management.

6. **Organize Awareness Events**: Take the initiative to organize awareness events in your community to educate the public about CHF. These events can include informational sessions, guest speakers, health fairs, or fundraising activities. Collaborate with local healthcare providers, community organizations, and CHF support groups to make the events impactful and reach a broader audience.

7. **Educate Others**: Become an advocate by educating others about CHF. Utilize social media platforms, community gatherings, or workplace wellness programs to share information about the signs, symptoms, risk factors, and management of CHF. Provide resources and materials that raise

awareness and encourage individuals to seek timely medical attention.

8. **Engage with Healthcare Providers**: Actively participate in your healthcare journey by establishing open communication and a collaborative relationship with your healthcare providers. Ask questions, seek clarification, and discuss any concerns you may have regarding your CHF management. By being an informed and engaged patient, you contribute to your own well-being while also encouraging quality care.

9. **Support Research and Fundraising Efforts**: Support CHF research and fundraising initiatives by making donations to reputable organizations dedicated to heart health. These contributions can help fund research, promote awareness campaigns, and support programs that benefit individuals living with CHF.

10. **Advocate for Prevention and Early Detection**: Within your social groups and community, emphasize the significance of CHF prevention and early detection. Promoting frequent checkups, adopting a heart-healthy lifestyle, and raising knowledge of the risk factors for heart disease are all important.

Raising CHF awareness and helping those who have the condition can be accomplished with any effort, no matter how tiny. You contribute to a stronger and more encouraging environment for people with CHF and their loved ones by actively participating in these activities and acting as an advocate.

Final Words of Encouragement

Congestive Heart Failure (CHF) can be challenging to live with, but it doesn't define you or prevent you from leading a purposeful life. Keep in mind that you are not traveling alone. There is a group of people, medical personnel, and support systems prepared to stand by your side.

Adopt a bold attitude as you negotiate the ups and downs of CHF, relying on your inner strength and the assistance of those around you. Learn about CHF, adhere to your treatment schedule, and place a high priority on self-care. Accept resiliency, confront fear head-on, and overcome challenges with tenacity.

Connect with organizations that are focused on CHF, attend support groups, and ask your loved ones for assistance. Share your experience and promote understanding and constructive change. By doing this, you can improve not only your own life but also the lives of others going through comparable difficulties.

Celebrate each success along the way, no matter how minor. Be hopeful, optimistic, and future-oriented. It is possible to manage CHF and have a full life because to improvements in research, available treatments, and the assistance of your healthcare team.

Consider each day as an opportunity to put your relationships, wellbeing, and health first. Adopt a balanced lifestyle, select healthy habits, and build resilience. Remember that you are more powerful than you might believe, and that you can live a life that is full of meaning and joy if you have the strength and tenacity to do so.

Never stop going forward, keep in touch with your network of supporters, and never forget the great strength you possess. You have the ability to live fearlessly despite having congestive heart failure and can overcome every obstacle that stands in your way.

I wish you fortitude, fortitude against adversity, and for a future of health, happiness, and fulfillment.

www.ingramcontent.com/pod-product-compliance
Lightning Source LLC
Chambersburg PA
CBHW061627250726

48659CB00004B/1114